The Perfect Doctor

•

forty voices on the imperfect pursuit of an ideal

ALSO BY PAGER PUBLICATIONS, INC.

—

in-Training: Stories from Tomorrow's Physicians
Family Doc Diary: A Resident Physician's Reflections in Fifty-Two Entries
in-Training: Stories from Tomorrow's Physicians, Volume 2
Salve: Words For The Journey
The Doctor Will Be Late
in-Training: 2020 In Our Words
Girl In A Bowtie: Lessons of a Pediatric Resident

The Perfect Doctor

•

forty voices on the imperfect pursuit of an ideal

edited by
Sasha Yakhkind, MD

foreword by Gordon Harper, MD
cover art by Sapana Adhikari, MD

PAGER PUBLICATIONS, INC.
a 501c3 non-profit literary corporation

The Perfect Doctor:
Forty Voices on the Imperfect Pursuit of an Ideal
edited by Sasha Yakhkind, MD

Copyright © 2024 by Pager Publications, Inc.. All rights reserved.

Published by Pager Publications, Inc. at pagerpublications.org.

Printed in the United States of America.

No part of this book may be used or reproduced in any manner whatsoever without written permission from Pager Publications, Inc., except in the case of brief quotations with proper reference embodied in critical articles and reviews.

All patient names, protected health information, and any other identifying information in this book have been changed to protect patient privacy.

Cover art by Sapana Adhikari.
Book design by Ajay Major.

First Printing: 2024

ISBN-13: 979-8-218-41601-0

To our teachers, who come in many different forms.

Contents

•

Pager Publications, Inc. Mission Statement — x
Foreword • Gordon Harper — xi
Introduction • Sasha Yakhkind — xiii

Premedical Perfection — 1

Take My Advice • Blessed Sheriff — 3
Most Highly Recommended • Emil Chuck — 10
Inner Struggles • M. Daniela Orellana Zambrano — 13
The Short Coat with a University Emblem • Timothy Barreiro — 15
Nightmares • Mallory Evans — 22
Behind Closed Doors • Zachary Simpson — 24

The Journey — 29

I Was Not Her • Eve Makoff — 31
My Mirage of Meaning • Audrey Nath — 34
Learning to Attend • Kimberly Lee — 37
The Arc of a Smile • Jazbeen Ahmad — 40
Gift • Sheenie Ambardar — 42
Signs and Symptoms • Melinda Ginne — 44

Lessons from Patients 51

Ricochet • Ajibike Lapite 53
High Wire History • Melani Zuckerman 60
The Birth Plan • Andrea Eisenberg 63
Paradox • Soma Sengupta 67
The Redeemer • Jeffrey Millstein 68
Octavian Was His Favorite Emperor • Anna Böhler 71
A Comfortable Silence • Amisha Patel 74
Eyes That See • Anna Delamerced 76

Burnout 79

The Puck • Joanne Wilkinson 81
Self-Care and Surgical Training • Rebecca Lynn Williams-Karnesky 84
Tethered • Harika Kottakota 88
Silence • Sapana Adhikari 90
No Absences • Charlotte Grinberg 92
Do No Self-Harm • Palak Shah 95

Doctors as Patients 99

How You Failed Me • Maya Sorini 101
The Other Place • Danielle Wilfand 104
The Mortal Physician • Rachel Scheub 109
Above and Beyond • Susie Jiaxing Pan 112
The View from the Other Chair • Miriam Colleran 114
Practice Your Humanity • Rohan Bhat 117

Diversity and Ethics   121

A Neurologist Takes Paternity Leave • Vincent LaBarbera   123

Why I Want My Next Doctor to be a Foreign Medical Graduate • Robert Lamb   127

A Good Doctor • Mayra Montalvo   130

The Best Doctors Stay Awake • Melissa Flanagan   132

Fading Photographs and Mournful Memories • Chinmayi Balusu   135

Immigrating Into Medicine • Pouya Ameli   138

Medicine Blinders • Alejandra Casillas   141

Secret Weapon • Chidinma Onweni   144

•

Afterword • John Sargent   146

References   148

Contributors   150

Acknowledgements   155

Pager Publications, Inc. Mission Statement

Pager Publications, Inc. is a 501c3 nonprofit literary organization
that curates and supports peer-edited publications
for the medical education community.

The organization strives to provide students and educators
with dedicated spaces for the free expression of their distinctive voices.

Pager Publications, Inc. was officially incorporated in January 2015
by its founders Ajay Major, Aleena Paul and Erica Fugger
to provide administrative and financial support for
in-Training and other publications.

Foreword

•

Medical humanities has come a long way, but the stories printed here represent a milestone in medical education for several reasons.

First, they give an authentic voice to students. Not voices echoing what faculty say or want to hear from students, or what students think faculty want to hear, nor echoes of the perfectionism to which students subject themselves. But these are voices that convey students' own experiences—their gratifying, exasperating, challenging, and rewarding experiences. The stories shared here are especially appreciated given how easy it can be for students to squelch their own voices, bowing to the demands of medical perfectionism. This is partly in response to the ways that medical training shakes up one's sense of self (Harper, 1993).

Second, these stories show how students, escaping from self-imposed (and maladaptive) perfectionism, can develop realistic expectations of themselves and others. This is a change in how one thinks of a person, from *the-way-he-is-and-always-will-be* to *he's-a-certain-way-now*. Such a change is a shift from what's called *essentialism* to a perspective of continuous *growth, learning, and healing*. Such a way of thinking helps not only when applied to oneself but also when applied to patients.

Third, the stories reflect the complexity of thinking that emerges in medical training, from thinking in one channel to learning how to join the patient empathically and simultaneously think in different terms. This has been called "clinical binocularity" (Harper, 2013).

All of this breaks up the distorted reading of William Osler's "Aequanimitas" when it is taken to mean that the physician has no feelings—is untouched by the patient's experience. What Osler meant was that the physician can have feelings but is able to function clinically. Here we appreciate (as I suspect Osler did, too), the complexity, not the simplicity of what is going on in the doctor.

Institutionally, we medical faculty have a huge role in facilitating the growth and differentiation of the students. For instance, curriculum should include small groups in which students share their reflections (Branch, 1995). The experience of sharing and feeling understood obviously increases the chances that the students will, in the future, help their patients feel understood as well.

The power of feeling understood has been much celebrated, outside as well as in medicine. In an early example, Virgil in the Aeneid, written in the first century BCE, describes how Aeneas, after the Trojan War ended with the Fall of Troy, failed to find solace elsewhere in the Mediterranean before staggering ashore in North Africa after his ship wrecked there. His loneliness and fear were abated when he saw, on the road to Carthage, a mural depicting, sympathetically, Priam escaping from Troy. "En Priamus," he said, "hic mentem mortalia tangunt et lacrimae rerum sunt." *Seeing Priam, it's clear that human suffering is noticed here; tears are shed for what we have endured.* Thus, sensing the possibility of feeling understood, Aeneas overcomes his fears and embarks on a history-making romance with Dido. As with Aeneas, feeling understood can be healing for all of us.

To all the student authors, thank you! And best wishes in your careers.

    Gordon Harper, MD
    Professor of Psychiatry, Harvard Medical School •

Introduction

•

Does the perfect doctor exist? In 2021, a group of fellows and new attendings from across the U.S. sat around a table at an Italian restaurant in Chicago after a long day of professional conferencing and discussed their experiences in training. A theme emerged: They all hid away parts of themselves to fit into the medical establishment, to be perfect. They were driven by family, role models, peers and almost always by their own dogged pursuit of an ideal. That's what you want your doctor to be, right? Someone who strives to be perfect. Or do you?

In the process of chasing perfection, these doctors forgot, lost, or let go of a core part of themselves. While these conflicts are not unique to medicine, the duration and intensity of training, and subsequent delay of development of life skills, lead to a particular kind of isolation from pre-medical core values. Many doctors come out of training with their brains filled with knowledge, but their souls drained of who they once were and what brought them to medicine in the first place. Some have been asked to cover up their tattoos, uncover their hair, wear heels, not wear heels, and dress according to their assigned sex. Many doctors have lived away from family for years. Even the young doctors who held onto their passions through medical school missed important milestones like holidays, weddings, and funerals in residency.

For some, it began when they were young. They loved art, but their immigrant parents insisted that medicine, law, and engineering were the only viable career paths. *I guess I'm good at science*, they told themselves, only later to feel out of place as the only creative in a sea of rote memorizers. Others wanted to do good, to save the world, then discovered corruption at the root of even the most selfless endeavors and settled for a comfortable, well-paid life. Some only knew about health care from their doctor parents' dinner conversations (or lack thereof) and didn't think about what makes *them* happy. For others, the competitive nature of pre-med classes led them to put their other interests aside to keep up. Others delayed having a family and then struggled to balance parenthood with the demands of medicine.

On my first day of medical school, a speaker told our class that medicine is not just a job, but that henceforth it has become our identity. The exact advice was along the lines of, "Next time you want to dance on the bar, think twice. You're representing your profession." In residency, I didn't have time to dance on bars, let alone much else other than to eat, sleep, and work. Medicine became my identity through the sheer amount of time I put into it. I felt stripped of what made me, me. I couldn't hold a reasonable conversation with people outside of medicine and worst of all, I lost the ability to meaningfully connect with patients and loved ones alike. I was burnt out.

My first years out of training were aimed at rediscovering my humanity. Through this book, conversations with friends, and increased media attention on burnout in health care, I have found that I am not alone.

•

Can medical students and doctors express their true identities and still be good doctors? I strongly believe the answer is yes. When you look at a stage full of eager first year medical students at their white coat ceremony, a sea of color literally turns to white as they don their coats. I wouldn't go as far as to say that the white coat ceremony should be abolished, but more attention needs to be paid to the colors and textures underneath. The cultural background, gender, affect, dress, tattoos and the way doctors express themselves are central to their identity. These core parts of themselves help patients as much as their approximation of encyclopedic knowledge. A patient may connect to her physician because they both wear hijabs and may open up parts of her history that would otherwise remain hidden. Another patient may see their doctor's rainbow flag tattoo and feel safe. A doctor can bond with a patient over marathon running, their children, or their own experience with disease. A doctor in mourning over the loss of themselves can't connect with patients, build trust, and offer the care that patients deserve.

Can doctors reach this type of holistic perfection while still building the technical expertise that is fundamental for their jobs? On the one hand, they must speak the same language of anatomy, physiology, and pharmacology to decipher the human body, treat disease and talk to each other. On the other hand, language is a communication tool and not an identity.

Through the personal stories of doctors, and some by those who work with them, this book argues that perfection has as many expressions as there are people. Medical students and doctors recount times that they came up against themselves, mentors, patients, and life circumstances to learn how they can be better doctors by being truer to themselves. Also included are eloquent perspectives of patients, other health care professionals, and a pre-medical school advisor who oversees the stringent and fraught selection process of future doctors. The book is broken down into six sections: the student perspective, the journey from becoming to being a doctor, lessons from patients, lessons from burnout, stories of doctors as patients, and a section on how diversity and ethics play into perfection.

The first section includes six stories about student struggles with perfection. One student writes about how the efficiency of medical rounds contradicted his values of connecting with patients in a meaningful way. A new student surprises himself with how he helped a patient, despite not fitting the typical doctor mold.

In the second section, six attendings share how their journeys through training and into professional life shaped who they are now. One doctor describes how, at every stage of her training, she was taught to question her assumptions. Another learned it was okay to smile, even though her training environment discouraged it. One doctor shares how her brother's death motivated her into medicine for the wrong reasons, only later to reconnect her with the deeper meaning behind their connection.

In the third section, doctors share what they learned from patients. There is a touching tale of a mother learning about her child's diagnosis with Rhett's syndrome, a debilitating disease characterized by seizures and developmental regression. The reader can see every movement of the doctor through the mother's eyes. This section includes two poems about coming up against the limitations of medicine in the face of expectations. It includes stories about patients who dispel generalizations that doctors learn at school, and instead teach them about life.

Section four is about burnout. It includes a poem and a painting by our cover artist. Every contribution to this section reflects on how training and work affected the writer, and how they took steps to find balance and reclaim what makes them human.

The fifth section has three stories and two pieces of artwork about doctors whose own illnesses played into their career and motivation. In one, a medical student writes a letter to a physician who treated her unkindly. Another describes how illness can make a physician feel like they belong and feel out of place at the same time. Another student envisions how the ideal doctor she would want to have is the same one she would want to be.

The last section is about the importance of diversity in medicine, and how ethical principles can guide practice and shape the field. One doctor reflects on how she did not appreciate what a patient really needed because she could not see past the blinders of her profession. A scientist recounts the barriers faced by foreign medical graduates in the United States. It takes another physician everything she has to smile in the face of prejudice.

Each story includes three to five questions for thought and discussion to stimulate the reader's own ideas. These are intentionally called "thought questions" and not discussion questions, because they can be answered by the individual reader in their minds or on paper, through discussion with peers, or in the classroom. Some of these stories may provoke strong emotions or disagreement. The goal of these questions is to prompt the reader to look inside to where their own reactions come from, to encourage their articulation, and maybe even to inspire their own writing!

One of my favorite words is *hysteresis*. It's used mostly in engineering to describe a response that depends on the timing or amount of stimulus. For example, a rubber band is easier to stretch after it's already been stretched, and alveoli in the lungs are easier to inflate once some volume of air is already inside of them. Hysteresis applies to culture change in medicine, too. Once research shows that a commonly held belief is harmful, initial change in practice faces more resistance than subsequent change after a movement has gained momentum. It has taken years for the ICU Liberation bundle, an evidence-based practice aimed at getting critically ill patients better faster, to overcome the outdated practice of oversedation (Ely, 2021). Research has shown repeatedly that burnt out, tired, overworked doctors and nurses are bad for health care, but doctors are still being asked to see more patients in less time (National Academy of Medicine, 2019). This book is one of the many efforts aimed towards a healthier health care system by giving its essential workers a voice.

My hope is that these stories move readers, motivate discussion, and spark change in individual lives, classrooms and workplaces. It is a call for trainees, medical schools, and hospitals to recognize the value of personhood as the underpinning of any academic, patient care, and financial mission. That requires time for students, residents, fellows and attending doctors to attend to personhood through reflection and adaptation. Every medical school and hospital's approach is going to look different, but one way to start is to listen to the voices of students and caregivers. That's what we're taught in medical school, right? That the patient's story holds the diagnosis? The esteemed neurologist José Biller once said something along the lines of, *if you don't know the diagnosis after taking the patient's history, take it again.*

It is worth noting that opinions expressed are those of the authors and do not represent the perspectives of their employers or institutions. Permission has been obtained from individuals referenced by name. Otherwise, names and details have been changed to protect the identity of patients and individuals described in these stories. I hope that you enjoy these stories as much as I did, and that they move all of us forward.

Sasha Yakhkind, MD
Tufts University School of Medicine •

Premedical Perfection

·

the student perspective

Take My Advice

•

Blessed Sheriff

"Open her legs."

I glared at daylight beaming through the fourth-floor window of the resident work room, announcing another day for the morning joggers outside the hospital window. For a flash of a moment, I allowed myself to daydream a version of myself floating down onto the sidewalk next to them. My momentary escape was interrupted by the sharp tapping of freshly painted vermilion nails which caught the first streaks of sunlight and reflected them back at me with peculiar urgency. A belligerent reminder to return my attention to my patient—or rather the tangled collection of notes, labs, and orders glowing from my laptop screen. The nails belonged to our senior resident and team leader, a fourth-year cardiology-hopeful with earnest eyes and an almost glossy precision that commanded authority and demanded deference.

"Open her legs." She repeated, sounding bored, but somehow angry.

"Huh?" I winced in confusion.

"Next time you go to examine her, open her legs. That's where the rash is."

"Okay," I mouthed, too embarrassed to apologize for missing yet another obvious symptom in our latest string of emergency room admits.

She nodded and returned to her desk, typing furiously. The acrylic wafting up from her nail polish forced a bitter smell into the air. Only thirty minutes into the day and she had managed to finish charting for all my assigned patients.

"Oh and let me know when you're ready for feedback. I have some advice."

I nodded weakly. Returning to my laptop screen, I attempted to hide my surprise. *Was it already time for midterm evaluations?* I had been so busy berating myself for barely keeping up with the rest of the team that I hadn't even thought to mentally prepare myself for the terrifying thought that soon my inadequacy might be formally confirmed. I felt my neck muscles tense in preparation for all the ecstatic nodding I was going to have to do in response to the oncoming litanies of "you're-doing-well-but-" and "you'd-be-just-fine-if-"

A reminder flashed across my screen, momentarily distracting me from the well of anxiety growing in my chest. It was almost time for morning didactics. I breathed a quick sigh of relief and quickly excused myself from the room.

Morning didactics were ostensibly protected learning time—but in reality, they were a golden opportunity for ten bleary-eyed medical students to frantically polish off their notes before morning rounds. We only half glanced at the Zoom screen in front of us where a graying doctor would describe the intricacies of some obscure disease process we would see maybe twice in our entire careers. It was a thrilling moment of freedom for me to be surrounded by the few people in the hospital who—like me—never quite understood what the fuck was going on and why it was all happening so fast. Of course, there were the geniuses among us, those who could list off a comprehensive differential diagnosis based off a headache and a single a bloody cotton swab—but the vast majority of us radiated a familiar angst from the same pit of confusion where all early-career physicians hide their most worn-out question: *Am I good enough at this?*

I found myself practically skipping to the tiny office at the back corner of the hospital where I discovered my fellow peers yawning a good morning to one another before the chorus of frenzied typing could begin. I ran through the list of patients in my head, attempting to exhaust the potential catalog of questions my team could ask during rounds. I almost got through the entire roster, flying through notes with a speed that surprised me. *What was Mr. Johnson's white blood cell count this morning? 17k. Could that represent a new infection in the absence of fever or other symptoms? What about Mrs. Gonzalez's recent urine culture which showed presence of bacteria? What was the drug of choice for complicated UTI again? And what about—*"Ms. Brown!" I exclaimed, involuntarily exposing my ramblings to the entire room.

I received a few worried glances before the chorus of typing continued, unabashed by my outburst. I managed to breathe a quick apology before tripping over myself into the hallway and onto the elevator. As the elevator slowly rumbled its way down to the patient ward, I silently scolded myself for skipping over Ms. Brown. She was my favorite patient and also my most... emotional. She often went on a long diatribe about almost anything: her family, a stranger, her past, her present, the nurses, her favorite book, her least favorite food, *anything*. I had gotten in the habit of seeing her first thing in the morning so I could ensure I had time to listen politely—why not? Sometimes the stories were entertaining, and I could tell she needed someone to talk to. Despite being here longer than any of my other patients, she hadn't received any visitors and, for some reason, that deeply bothered me. Maybe it was because she looked so much like my own mother who I had left alone, 300 miles away, so I could go to medical school.

This morning was the exception. I decided on a whim that I would save Ms. Brown for last, as a new patient had been admitted the night before and I needed a thorough history. However, in the fogginess of twilight on little sleep, it had slipped my mind to circle back on Ms. Brown. Now—I jostled my phone out of my pocket to check the time—I had less than *ten minutes* to see her before morning rounds started. I reminded myself to breathe, and secretly hoped she would be asleep when I entered the room, too drowsy for her usual conversation.

"Well *there* you are," I heard a jovial voice call from a mountain of bleached sheets. I entered the room smiling, despite myself.

"Good morning, Ms. Brown," I called back, resisting the urge to ask her how she was doing—lest she launch into a passionate breakdown of the morning's events. I made my way to her bedside and began our normal routine. *Any pain? Trouble sleeping? Medications still working okay?* Simultaneously, I took quick notes on any physical changes in her appearance from the night before, observing her fluid status, heart rate, and blood pressure as I felt for her pulses. A quick abdominal exam and a moment listening to her heart and lungs, and I would be on my way out. In disbelief, I rubbed the bell of my stethoscope, thanking the heavens that time was on my side.

I pressed the diaphragm of my stethoscope to her chest only to hear the muffled vibration of a voice blocking what should have been the clear *da-dum* rhythm of a heartbeat. Cautiously I removed my right earpiece, "What was that, Ms. Brown?" I asked.

"I said, you ever heard this song?" She held up a small phone screen and I had to squint to read the small print written below a vintage album cover.

"Open My Heart... by Yolanda Adams," I read aloud. She nodded slowly. "Never heard it," I said nonchalantly, slipping my earpiece back in and attempting once more to listen to her heart. In truth I *had* heard it—about a million times every Sunday morning of my childhood. It was an old gospel favorite of my mother and I had it memorized word for word. But I didn't need to have a conversation about it now.

"*Talk to me mhmm talk to me...*" I heard the first notes of the song playing loudly over Ms. Brown's speaker. She bobbed her head along to the soulful melody, and I could tell she was about to start singing. Defeated, I removed my stethoscope from her chest and begrudgingly watched her sing the first few lines of the song, willing her to pick up the tempo so I could listen for her lung sounds and maybe call it a day.

Alone in a room, just me and yoOUU

The familiar lyrics washed over me like a flood.

I'm all burned out
And I don't think my strength's gonna last
So I'm crying out
Crying out to you
Lord I know that you're the only one
Who is able to pull me through

When she finished the last few lines of the verse, I could see the corners of her eyes crinkle with confusion and a little bit of sadness. All of a sudden, the room was silent. Relieved at first, I reached for my stethoscope... but sensing another kind of opportunity in the quiet, instead I found myself reaching for her hand. After a few minutes, she started up again, singing almost entirely through the final chorus.

"You have a beautiful voice, Ms. Brown," I offered, watching her wipe away a few stray tears.

"Thank you, baby," she said, a smile beginning to lift the corners of her lips. "I used to sing all the time. But this world... sometimes you forget how good the Lord is. You know something? When I first got here, after a while, I didn't have no hope. Always being in pain, always alone. You don't know really know how alone you can be. When my husband died, that's when I knew. Not having someone looking out for you all the time. Just someone to listen to. Someone to trust. But I'm starting to look forward to going home, now I know someone out there might miss the sound of my voice in the morning." An inexplicable pang of emotion shot through me.

"That's right. And we're going to get you feeling better so you can—"

"Excuse me," a voice called urgently from the doorway.

My senior resident strode confidently into the room. She nodded in greeting to Ms. Brown who smiled back and said hello. My face flushed with embarrassment realizing it was nearly time for morning rounds, and not only had I not yet submitted half of my notes, I had also been caught skipping the morning didactic. This was going to be a very interesting midterm evaluation.

"Excuse me," I heard again, this time directly in front of me. With mortification, I realized I was still holding tightly to Ms. Brown's hand, blocking my senior resident from examining the patient. I stepped back quietly and watched as she deftly collected an interval history and completed a quick cardiopulmonary exam in what felt like mere seconds. Ms. Brown still looked teary eyed, but I could tell she didn't have any more conversation in her, making it easier to quickly file out of the room behind my senior resident.

"Don't worry about presenting this patient," she mumbled, staring straight ahead. "I know you didn't get to do a full exam." I let out a breath I didn't know I'd been holding.

"Also, are you ready for your feedback?"

"Sure," I said a little too eagerly.

Without another word she took a sharp right, leading me into the same conference room where didactics were usually held. On the board I could see the chicken scratch handwriting of the doctor who had attempted to teach us about cardiomyopathies. Dutifully, I pulled out notepad and pen and waited for her to begin.

"What do you feel like you have done well here over the past few weeks?" she started.

With feigned confidence I told her about how I was beginning to feel more comfortable with physical exams and how I felt my presentations had been slowly improving. Her facial expression remained blank, but in the back of my mind I couldn't help but think she was itching to disagree. Instead, she moved on to another question.

"And what do you think you still need to work on?"

"Well... I suppose I'm having issues with time management. I always feel like I'm in a rush to see everyone and do everything I'm supposed to. You know?" I felt it was better to get it out onto the table now so that she wouldn't have to bring it up. I took her vigorous nodding as proof that she accepted my assessment and, as expected, her tone became sterner.

"Yes, and I do expect you to participate *fully* in morning didactics." Her eyes narrowed as she glanced somewhere beyond me. "It's important that you are present. It reflects poorly on your team when you are distracted elsewhere," she sighed. "And on this point, I have some advice you'd be smart to take. What time do you arrive to the hospital?"

I blinked, confused at the question. "Typically, the medical students arrive by 6 a.m.," I answered.

She sat back in her chair, arms crossed. "You should be arriving earlier than that. When I was in medical school, I got here around 5 a.m."

I swallowed hard. *I guess there goes another hour of sleep I didn't have. But if that's the worst of it...*

"And another thing." Her demeanor seemed to soften slightly, and this time she looked me in the eye, with a slightly pained expression. "You're quite difficult to approach." I could tell by the way she cleared her throat that this conversation was veering into uncomfortable territory for both of us.

"By difficult, I mean... well... I'm worried that you feel things very deeply. Sometimes I look at your face, and I feel that you're almost... emotional?"

Oh no. This can't be happening.

"It's a lot of... sensitivity. I've noticed this in your interaction with patients as well." I instantly cringed thinking about what must have gone through her mind when she saw me holding Ms. Brown's hand. *Was I being unprofessional?*

"I don't mean to say you shouldn't empathize with patients. I'm rather concerned about your efficiency. You have a lot to do, and you have to develop a better rhythm and control over the day-to-day demands. Do you understand?"

I nodded yes, feeling embarrassed, but not quite understanding why. I tried to suppress the heat rising to my cheeks, which would be an inappropriate giveaway that I was yet again emotional. Reflexively, I flashed back through all feedback I had ever received from other senior doctors.

Had any of them seen in me the same dreaded sentimentality? Was I too easy to read? An awkwardly open book of "inefficient" emotions and feelings? And did it really make me "difficult" to work with?

THE PERFECT DOCTOR

Before I could let my musings throw me into a spiral, I busied myself tucking away my notebook and pen. Slowly, and with calculated stoicism, I rose to thank my senior resident for her feedback. Together we rejoined the rest of our team in the adjacent work room for morning rounds.

And I tried. Despite my best efforts, I couldn't let go of my new emotional self-consciousness. When it was time for me to present my patients, I kept track of every body movement, every adjective, and every tone shift. I did my best to emulate my senior resident with a fixed facial expression and short matter-of-fact statements. When I told my team about Mr. Johnson's white blood count, I resisted mentioning his newfound infectious joy now that speech had finally approved him to eat solid foods. When I recounted Mrs. Gonzalez's UTI symptoms, I reduced her ache, fatigue, and a new bathroom phobia down to simple dysuria. I didn't tell them that I found out Ms. Brown could sing. Or what I had found out about her husband. The new attitude felt sharper—more economical, but also exhausting. What kind of doctor doesn't *feel*?

I feared the inevitable confrontation with Ms. Brown during afternoon rounds and rehearsed how I could move past the emotions and do medicine instead. I practiced a curt greeting all the way down the elevator, and an equally efficient farewell for the evening.

I was going to do this. I was on my way to becoming a better doctor.

This time when I entered the room, she was peacefully sleeping. The remnants of her lunch rested precariously on the edge of the tray table in front of her. I quickly took note of her condition, got an update from the nurse in the room, and was on my way out when I noticed her lunch tray tipping over.

"Shoot!" I whispered, managing to just barely push the tray back onto the table while generating a noisy stirring from Ms. Brown's bed.

"Doctor?"

I paused and smiled briefly. "Hey there, Ms. Brown, just doing a quick check-in. However, you should know I'm not a doctor yet. Give me about…" I pretended to check my watch. "…14 more months."

She smiled incredulously, "Really? Could've fooled me. You let me know when you open your practice, I'll be your first patient!"

The exhaustion of the day suddenly melted from my shoulders as her words of affirmation sliced through the emotional void I had been perfecting all day. "Thank you, Ms. Brown, I really—I deeply appreciate you."

She continued. "You know what would make this place better?" She gestured vaguely to the bland hospital walls surrounding us. "People who care. I don't have many people around, but I know you're looking out for me. That has made this all easier. *That* means the world."

I searched her face for a moment, and instantly knew her words were true. And though unsolicited, her confession felt, to me, the best advice I had received all day. Suddenly, and as a matter of principle, I remembered whose evaluation mattered most.

Of all the things I had to accomplish in a day, my final and best achievement would always be listening for the heart. And not just to hear it beat. But also, to hear it laugh, cry, rant, dream, and be that most human of all organs. You can't move past your humanity to do medicine. And medicine had no right to make me any less kind.

Without checking to see if anyone was watching, I took Ms. Brown's hand in mine. "I'll see you first thing tomorrow morning."

She smiled. "Goodbye, doctor." •

Thought questions:
- Who is the better doctor: the resident or the student? Why?
- What needs to change to allow for efficiency and connection to patients?
- What would have happened to Ms. Brown were it not for this student?

THE PERFECT DOCTOR

Most Highly Recommended

•

Emil Chuck

"The elephant is a very large animal," said the Rajah kindly. "Each man touched only one part. Perhaps if you put the parts together, you will see the truth."
—The Blind Men and the Elephant

The journey of a physician begins with an application. The applicant shows a personal roadmap of their drive to pursue medicine as a career. Mileposts are documented: educational circumstances before college, pre-professional course grades, highlights of significant experiences, and a personal introduction to the screeners who will review the application.

The admissions committees I've served on involve many people who look at different parts of an application in isolation, like the blind sages describing an elephant to the Rajah. One person makes a judgment on grades. Another looks at community service. Another looks at interview feedback. Each person carries a perspective and an expectation for what would pass muster. When everyone's input is accounted for, the holistic process presumes that the picture of the true applicant and future physician emerges. Within the crucible of file deliberation, the preferences of individual committee members are debated and "averaged" to establish some precedent examples and help select our next class.

Over my years as an advisor and an admissions counselor, many aspiring doctors have highlighted their achievements as competency badges. Shadowing three different doctors in outpatient, in-patient, or community care settings somehow is not enough. They push themselves to appeal to admissions committees, so they show they can put a lot on themselves and still come out with 4.0 grade point averages (GPA), 98th percentile exam results, and impact as a community change agent. All this effort is to be desirable to "top 20" U.S. News and World Report medical school programs. According to many students, anything less than getting into these brand-name schools could disappoint their families.

We want an excellent class in all possible ways: academic achievement, social impact, creative ability, interpersonal savvy, and a sense of professionalism that goes beyond satisfying requirements. Through stellar grades and strong mentoring, each should have little trouble with preclinical exams or clinical experiences. Every member should be adaptable and resilient to all the changes that come with medical education, with different professors, mentors, and preceptors shaping the different facets of each "elephant" that they touch. The desirable medical student represents all the ideal characteristics and competencies as well as the high GPA and Medical College Admission Test (MCAT) scores to boost our medical school's perceived reputation as a quality program. As our program leadership says, excellence and diversity are not mutually exclusive goals. Each class must have both and be better than last year's class in every way.

All the applicants' letters of recommendations deem them to be "most highly recommended." They are flawless, highly motivated, and competent in the author's eyes. One candidate has a letter from a research professor with whom the candidate presented three posters and is in line for an author's contribution to a future paper. The data collected by the applicant should help with a future grant proposal for the professor, and, unfortunately, the student will leave the lab for medical school. "Most highly recommended ... one of the best students I have had in 30 years." But has the professor really had time to truly mentor this student, or was this task left to various postdocs and graduate students as the pressure to get the grant builds? Tenure does not reward mentoring students at most institutions. A different professor knows the student from lecture classes, from the cavernous introductory weed-out course to the more conversational discussion class with 20 other students. They are "most highly recommended" because the student engaged with the material and asked thoughtful questions. This professor describes a dozen such students in this way every cycle.

The letters are remarkably similar, as if following a template akin to Mad Libs. A letter from a clinician that the applicant shadowed for about 20 hours states, "The student was punctual, well-prepared, courteous, and willing to listen to others. "Most highly recommended" again. A different letter from a physician with whom this applicant worked 1000 hours as a medical assistant: "most highly recommended." The food pantry supervisor was just as effusive.

The admissions committee admitted this particular student along with a full-ride scholarship. Within two years, the student was dismissed, saying medicine "just wasn't right for me." None of the letters hinted at the problems we experienced with this student before dismissal. This happens with a handful of students who fail to be promoted every year.

Every faculty screener wonders where they missed the signs of failure. Even when they have high grades and scores, why don't they still perform up to our expectations? Even with multiple mini-interview (MMI) questions and situational judgment exams for predoctoral and residency selection, students still have professionalism issues despite being "most highly recommended." Many faculty members are frustrated with the lack of certainty in selecting future physicians. Students spiral into self-doubt and wonder if they could ever be the consoling, empathetic idealistic premed student they were only a few years ago. Physicians and health care workers experience more exhaustion and burnout. And a thousand inspirational quotes on leadership, perfection, success, and competency ring hollow to so many who feel that their vision of being a doctor has become more of a nightmare.

Does being "most highly recommended" confer a false sense of confidence to the inevitable challenges of being a medical student and a physician? Does every student fall from the pedestal, and some take the fall better than others? It is not only the student, but society that expects doctors to be perfect. Perhaps this unrealistic expectation is the elephant in the room that we can only see if we talk about it and work together. •

Thought questions:
- What could soften the fall from "most highly recommended" to the realities of becoming a doctor?
- Should medical school applicants be open about their personal challenges? If so, is there a limit to how open applicants should be?
- If applicants do bear all, how does someone on the admissions committee curb their own implicit biases surrounding applicants' authenticity and perceived imperfection?

Inner Struggles

•

M. Daniela Orellana Zambrano

As first-year medical students in Ecuador, my best friend and I used to daydream about what types of doctors we would become. We were highly motivated and enthusiastic about our medical careers, but always wondered how we would be when "we grew up." We aspired to be the best doctors for our patients. Although we didn't know what that entailed, we found some answers from the doctors we met along the way. We would play, choosing features we admired the most from each of our professors. I remember we said something along the lines of "I would like to be an excellent educator and challenge students as our biology professor does, but as understanding and personable as our biostatistics professor. As involved with our patients as our family medicine preceptor, and as smart and knowledgeable as our neurology professor." We were confident that putting all those pieces together would be the recipe for success.

The time to be one of them finally came. As a medical intern in the United States, I was ready to work and practice like those I admire.

The first days as an intern were filled with new roles and scenarios, first impressions, and racing thoughts. One day after seeing my patients, I kept thinking of our conversations. Mr. S had not had any more episodes of emesis, which was great, but I noticed he was in a low mood. *I should have asked him more about it.* An MRI showed a brain tumor in one of my patients, and I had to break the news. That was my first time doing so. I couldn't help but wonder how that went. *I should have stayed with them longer, giving them time to process.*

During rounds, my attending asked me about fever as I presented my patients. I missed that critical piece of information. The patient I wanted to discharge had a fever, and I didn't even realize it. *I am doing a terrible job*, I thought. Where was my patient going after discharge? I didn't know; I forgot to read the social work notes. *I can't be making these kinds of mistakes four months into intern year. My senior must think I am an absolute mess. I wonder if he would trust me with the care of his patients. I am not the doctor I thought I would become. I am nothing close to the attendings I had always looked up to.*

To know it all, to see it all, to do it all. Those are expectations for myself, and the inevitable failure to achieve them frustrates me, creating conflict that affects my relationships with my patients and coworkers. This idea of what I should be is misleading. It leaves me isolated, and I forget about the honor that is to be a doctor, to have another human being confide in you and rely on you to find them an answer.

Only if I accept where I am and work from there, with patience and humility, and not let pride get in the way, I could be a step closer to the doctor I would like to be. I have all the resources, excellent attendings, seniors, and co-interns that are only ready to help. But I have to start with myself. I am not where I would like to be, but that doesn't mean I won't ever get there.

As I write this, I am reliving the pain, the frustration, and the embarrassment; the only difference is that now I can tell that it comes from my own expectations. I aim to spend less time reliving the wrongs and more time moving forward in my daily life as an intern. •

Thought questions:
- What feelings come up when you remember a moment you failed?
- What techniques do you have to process those feelings?
- How do you help others overcome failure?

The Short Coat with a University Emblem

•

Timothy Barreiro

"Every particular in nature, a leaf, a drop, a crystal, a moment of time is related to the whole, and partakes of the perfection of the whole."
—Ralph Waldo Emerson

A cross from the emergency room was a small, six-bed extern house, the place medical students on clerkship rotations stayed. Clerkships, the clinical training years of medical students, often follow the first two years of intensive book reviews, scheduled didactics, never-ending lectures, and laboratory work. During clerkship years, students can rotate at different hospitals and in different specialties, such as cardiology or pulmonary medicine. All students anticipate clerkship, hoping for real patient interactions and the first sense that they are becoming a *real* doctor. Hospital medical students are easily identified by a short white coat with a university emblem on the arm or front pocket. All that knowledge from books behind them, clerkship is the time for real patient encounters.

For my first clerkship, I arrived the day before we were to start and checked in with security. My room assignment faced the emergency room entrance with lines of ambulances. The sounds of sirens were like the melody of chirping crickets. The first day's agenda was to meet in the auditorium for an overview of the hospital and to meet faculty and residents. I made a mental list: meeting at 7 a.m.; up a 5:30 a.m.; shower; tie, and short white coat with university emblem on the arm. Cross the emergency room parking lot, dodging ambulances. I had it all figured out. With nervous anticipation, I knew that tomorrow was going to be a great day.

I awoke to an orchestra of sirens and glanced over at the clock: 6:35 a.m. What the blank! No shower, makeshift tie, balled up short white jacket with university emblem on the arm, I was dodging ambulances like a Heisman trophy winning running back. I could make it. I would make it. As I dodged the last ambulance and hurdled the gurneys, the emergency room doors parted like the Red Sea of old. That is when I met Cletus.

Cletus was a thin, tall man, wearing overalls, just like I assumed he did every day of his farming life. His boots were caked with a clay mud mixture, both dry and wet. He donned a frayed worn John Deere hat, so faded you could hardly make out the typical green color. His insulated shirt was also worn at the ends, evidence of his occupation and hard work ethic. His wife, a gentle woman and similarly frail, was well kept. Appearing in her late 70s, she had striking gray-white hair, with just a speckle of black. She was standing over Cletus in the doorway and immediately came to me as I parted the sea.

"Please help us. He is in terrible pain. I think it is his stomach. I begged him for days, and he would not listen."

I cannot tell you how many times in my life I have heard those words from families. Cletus, I expected, was not a man to be bothered by subtle aches that came from a day in the fields.

Agh. What to do?

"Miss, I'm just a student."

"Please, he is in pain and cannot walk."

In that second, the world seemed slower. I looked around only to see a sea of ambulances. Inside, the emergency room hummed like a beehive: each bee with a unique purpose, dodging, flying around in various directions with imperfect perfection. I wondered how Cletus sat in pain in the emergency room entrance without anyone seeing him. As my focus came back to Cletus and his wife, I looked over to see a wheelchair. My first command medical decision: get a wheelchair. I could wheel him into the emergency room and run to the auditorium. *Still time*, I thought. *Still time.*

Cletus was in severe pain and curled up in the fetal position. Any subtle movement, even extending my arm to hold his elbow, elicited a face of fear and discomfort. Aided by his wife, we got Cletus into the wheelchair.

"Okay, doing well here," I said out loud, not sure if I meant that as a kind word to Cletus or to myself. Time was of the essence. Now, just get him to triage and run to the auditorium. Just as we start to move, Cletus, with his stern, heroic, but direct voice, said, "Thanks."

I give him a quick short smile, the kind that just lifts the corners of your mouth. *Keep moving*, I said in my internal voice. Then, like the Grand Inquisitors of the Galactic Empire, Cletus asked, "Doctor, what's causing my pain?"

I try to get words out, but they stuck. "I'm just a student," I replied, but Mrs. C followed with "Please just help him."

So, with all my medical expertise of the past hour, I did the only thing that just seemed medical: I placed my hand on his abdomen. I could feel the boom, Boom, BOOM of a mass in his stomach. Although I tried to reassure both Cletus and his wife, the expression on my face must have elicited shock. They both spoke with unity that comes with 50 years of marriage: "Is it bad?"

I may not have known much, but I knew it was not good. I suspected he had an abdominal aortic aneurysm (AAA), an enlargement and dilation of the major blood vessel that supplies blood to internal organs, including kidneys and intestines. The blood vessel called the abdominal aorta travels down the back, near the spine, and was likely the cause of his searing pain. The aorta, a large vessel extending off the heart, changes names from thoracic to abdominal aorta as it passes unique anatomical structures. The abdominal aorta then divides in the lower abdomen into vessels that supply the legs. I reached down to check the lower extremities; pulses were weak, indicating poor blood flow. At that second, a million images, impulses and a lecture flashed in my mind. My face must have relaxed, and I replied to them, "No, he will be okay."

In reality, I had no idea, but the one thing I did know: we needed help. Fast. I wheeled Cletus into the main area of the emergency room, past triage. Most hospital wards are the same. Surrounding the peripheries are hospital beds or rooms with a small central area, usually enclosed in glass, to provide privacy, called the fishbowl. In the fishbowl, staff, doctors, and care providers huddle to discuss, chart, and decipher issues in the ward. I approached this area with a sense of urgency. Yet, the symphony of a busy, hectic, scattered harmony did not stop.

"Hello. I need help. Hello. I need some help. We need some help here."

After what seemed to be an eternity, finally, I was answered by an athletically fit physician with auburn hair and a needed, welcoming smile. Dr. Laura, I learned later, was an emergency room attending.

"What ya need?" she replied, with a tone of confidence, experience, and comfort.

"I have Cletus. He was in the emergency room ambulance door hunched over..." Explanations came out like hot lava rupturing out of a volcano.

Dr. Laura to my surprise nodded and asked, "What ya think it is?" I started to say, stopped, then said, "I am a stu—." She cut me off in mid-sentence and expressed: "I know you are a student, but I want to know what you think."

Wow, really. Okay. "I think he has a triple A that is rupturing." With a certain flair and yet nurturing nature, we were in movement. As I looked around, there were now at least two nurses, Cletus, and his wife in a room, on a gurney. Vital signs were being completed.

"What would you do then to confirm this?" Dr. Laura asked.

"Hum, not sure. A CT scan but maybe a quick look with ultrasound."

"Good," she replied. "Let's do the ultrasound right now, and depending on what we see, we can then get the CT."

An ultrasound probe was placed on Cletus' abdomen. He was feeling less pain after the administration of morphine. Dr. Laura explained the procedure as it was being performed in a timeless, effortless, simultaneous unity to which I would soon get accustomed, as an experienced physician learns to save previous time and effort. A thin sheet of gel was laid across the abdomen.

"A little cold, Mr. Smith."

Ultrasound was not new to me. I understood the device and had seen images before. But a unique world appeared with clarity. It seemed like a new universe being explored. The image still illuminates my mind, like it happened just yesterday. Most physicians remember specific people, places, and events, like this one. We tell stories and jokes about these events to alleviate pain and to bond us as a band of brothers.

Dr. Laura stated, looking over at the nurse. "Let's call vascular surgery and get a CT scan with runoff." Just as Cletus and his wife were about to ask a question, she looked up and pointed to the ultrasound screen.

"Mr. Smith, as the young doctor stated, it appears you have an aneurysm or enlargement of the artery near your stomach. If it ruptures, you could be in severe danger."

Mrs. Smith's words were simply elegant. "Oh, my."

Events moved in absolute stillness. "Oh no," I said. "What time is it?"

"7:35 a.m. Why?"

"I was to be in the auditorium at seven."

"You'd better hurry."

I left Cletus and his wife without a word or goodbye. I ran to the next objective, forgetting what had just happened. I opened the doors of the auditorium with one hand, while swinging my now unpressed short white coat with a university emblem over my shoulders. I entered a room, an alien world. Lines of white-coated students filled the front rows. Residents were sleeping and reading anything non-medical in the back rows. For the residents, this was time off, away from work. This was mandatory time with no responsibility, a time to rest. However, just a few rows down, sat medical students, sitting stiffly upright with clipboards in hand, and new fancy pens, graduation gifts for newly minted doctors.

The door of the auditorium slammed shut so loud, it sounded as if the horns of Odin bellowed throughout the hospital signaling *the stupid one has arrived*. As the blast echoed and pierced the auditorium, all the residents and medical students turned to look at me like a synchronized swim team.

"Nice of you to join us," came from the auditorium podium. I was not sure who made the statement. Feelings of anger, frustration, and embarrassment rushed within me so fast, I felt dizzy. In what felt like an eternity, I joined the back row of residents.

This is when I met Joe, the chief resident. Being elected chief resident is both an honor and privilege. The chief position is typically given to a graduating resident who fellow residents and faculty feel best represents a program. The concept of chief resident originated with William Halstead, chief surgeon at The John Hopkins Hospital in Baltimore in the late 1800s. Usually, the position is held for one year. Historically, the chief's role was controlling the operating and work schedule, thereby determining the experience to be gained by others. This hierarchical position within the educational system mandated respect and authority. Joe looked at me with a slight shock of disbelief and amazement. He leaned over and quietly, but firmly, said, "Maybe you should sit down in front."

At the time I was confused. Did he not want to be next to me because I was now on a panel of the administrators' top ten to watch list? I visualized the list with my picture plastered on the wall of the doctor's lounge allowing all attendings to track my every movement. Did Joe not want to be noticed near a student who could not make it to the first mandatory meeting on his first day of his first rotation on time? Guilt by association? I was now the new plague.

As I got up to move down with clerkship classmates, every step, turn, and movement was amplified by a thousand, like the sound floorboards make when you sneak around the house, trying hard not to wake a baby. Getting situated in the lower seats, I was lucky to sit next to Marne. Marne was from my medical school. She wore the same emblem on the side of her jacket. She was from the community, glad to be doing clerkship so close to her home. She could live at home and save money, get laundry done, and eat home-cooked meals. As I sat down and sank lower in my seat, she grinned at me with a chuckle. I leaned over, asking, "What part of the program are we on?"

"Professionalism," she replied with a witty smirk.

"Fantastic," I replied.

Soon after the overview and orientation, we moved on to selected rotations. I was on pulmonary medicine, a very demanding and rewarding rotation. We were asked to meet in the bronchoscopy suite, where we were going to meet our first patient. Bronchoscopy has become an integral part of pulmonary medicine. The procedure had begun before we entered the room. The patient was under conscious sedation, when a patient is placed into a tranquil sleeping state but is not so sedated that they need an oral or fixed airway, such as needed during an operation.

Dr. R was a brilliant bedside teacher and clinician. I loved that he treated the whole patient, even though his specialty was pulmonary and critical care. I was with Joe, the same resident who directed me in the auditorium, and who avoided me like the plague. Later, I learned that he was planning to do anesthesia after residency. The procedure was a bronchoscopy with biopsy. It involved a long flexible light wand advanced into the airways to examine lungs for abnormalities and a tiny scissors in the scope to obtain a biopsy if needed. As we entered the room, Joe whispered to me, "Are you ready?" Sure, I was ready. *Wait, ready for what?*

Dr R. was an exceptional attending with exquisite skills and knowledge. He was also a master at pimping. Pimping, a unique term in medicine popularized in 1989, has an origin dating to 17th century London. Robert Koch, the father of germ theory, had a series of pümpfragen that was commonly used on his teaching rounds. Pimping is a unique art. It has good and bad attributes. It is a rite of passage for medical students and residents. It started just as we entered the room. Questions came like a Gatling gun: rapid, never-ending, and loud—with precision hits to my confidence.

"What are the subsegments of the right upper lobe?"

"Who performed the first bronchoscopy?" "What is this?" "What is that?"

As I stuttered and stammered with each passing question, I don't even remember if I got any correct. I started to wonder. *Well, basket weaving looks like a good career.*

We moved on to the next patient on the respiratory ward. Chronic lungers with exacerbations of chronic obstructive airway disease (COPD). We examined patients and discussed treatment and diagnostic adjustments on each. Then, we broke to attend noon conference. Noon conference was when didactics, or formal lectures, occurred. They were subject-based and typically presented by an attending. The noon conference was on etiologies and care of the post-operative delirious patient. I wasn't post-operative, but I fit the delirious part well. With no real time to eat, we usually grabbed lunch in the hospital cafeteria and ate during lecture. Questions or pimping still occurred, depending on which attending was presenting lecture. Joe approached me at the end of the lecture.

"Dr. R wants us to meet him in operating room 1 for a closed pleural biopsy."

Commonly done in the past when tuberculosis was prevalent, Cope or Abrams closed pleural biopsies are rarely done anymore with the advent of video-assisted surgery and pleuroscopy. Both are invasive procedures that take small samples of tissue from the internal lining of the thorax called the parietal pleura. Diseases of the pleura are rare today. As we entered the operating room suite, Joe leaned towards me and whispered, "Don't touch anything." *Okay,* I replied.

The patient was sitting upright with arms extended up near his shoulders. He looked like he was doing a Russian Cossack dance without the squatting. We approached Mr. H. Dr. R explained to Mr. H that he was going to have to help with the procedure; the patient agreed. I approached the patient and introduced myself. I started to walk around back, to where OR staff had laid out key instruments for the procedure. All I kept thinking about was Joe telling me not to touch anything. But, like a moth to the flame, as I moved to the back of the patient, I tripped, hitting the instrument tray and knocking it over. Instruments with their pristine stainless steel shine tumbled over onto the floor, like a tumbleweed moving across a Western saloon town. "Oh shit," was the last thing I remember saying, as the biopsy needle bounced on the floor, like a kid in a giant bounce-a-round. After the initial eyes of amazement had glanced over me, we came to realize that the hospital only had one pleural biopsy tray. This one set would need to be re-sterilized. That would take about one hour. Dr. R apologized to Mr. H. The operating room team rearranged the schedule to allow us to conduct the procedure later.

The remaining day was a continued downward spiral of misadventures and mishaps. Among ten thousand questions, I got three correct. We finished notes. I went to the library to look up questions. When I looked at the clock, it was late. I decided it was time to head back to the extern house; tomorrow would be a new day. As I started to make my way out of the hospital, I heard a faint voice that kept getting louder.

"Doctor, Doctor."

I ignored it. I was just a student with a small white coat with a university emblem on the side.

However, by forces unknown to all of us, I turned around, only to see Mrs. Smith, Cletus's wife from the emergency room. She was more composed than I was, given the time of day and my derangement.

"Doctor, thank you!"

"What?" I replied.

"Thank you." She went on to explain that Cletus did have a partial rupture of an aneurysm and it got repaired. He was currently recovering in the surgical intensive care unit. Then, she gave me a great big hug, a never-ending, clenching, completely consuming grasp, like grabbing a large teddy bear that is so soft, you cannot imagine it is real. After additional thanks and formalities, I continued out of the hospital.

I wondered how I could have forgotten about the morning events in the emergency room. I had spent much of the day screwing things up. So much so that I wondered, was I in the right profession? Could I do this doctor thing? Was I made up for this type of work? I had spent so much time focusing on my errors, I was remiss in forgetting about a win. The events of Cletus ran through my mind the rest of the night. As I passed through the emergency room, out the door, dodging the ambulances coming in, I started to smile. *I can do this. I want to do this.*

Sometimes medicine and the culture that surrounds it makes it hard to see the human condition. We spend so much time trying to be a doctor, we lose sight of the personal connections that are bigger than the diagnosis. We all have insecurities, events that mold and affect our lives. We all have small daily challenges. At this point in my career, I realize now that being a physician is asymptotic: I try every day to be that person. A physician with titles, awards, or advanced degrees is less important than the person that provides hope and shows care. Physicians need to stop and recognize small wins and learn from our losses. Physicians need to remain humble, and be reminded that doing this profession is a privilege, not a right. It is about connections with other people and the patients with whom we talk. It is about interacting and sharing ourselves with others. Doing that and providing hope embodies the best of medicine. •

Thought questions:
- Is pimping a necessary form of teaching?
- How should educators most effectively help students and peers learn from mistakes?
- How should Dr. R have responded when the narrator knocked over the surgical tray?
- What emotions did you experience as you traveled with the author on their first day in the hospital?

THE PERFECT DOCTOR

Nightmares

•

Mallory Evans

I stand at the bedside with perfect clarity: lab values memorized, images read and interpreted, literature perused, primed with the next best step. I even remember choice anecdotes about the patient's life, prepared to demonstrate the perfect balance of sophisticated knowledge and friendly relatability. Infinite preparation for today's rounds was fit into a narrow window between ironing my pants, running 10 miles, and kissing my husband before leaving for work. I am the embodiment of well-roundedness, singularly devoted to medicine. I ask thoughtful questions. I nod my head, raise my eyebrows, smile with my eyes above the mask. There is no acne on my chin. My hair is shiny and full. I am humbly self-reliant. I don't pack lunches; I don't miss eating them. My curiosity is curated, my mind pruned from a winding maze to an inescapable funnel. There's nothing more important I could become than a physician. I go to bed at night, believing there's nothing more I could have done.

I wake up just past midnight, gasping.

Behind. The day hasn't even started, and I'm already behind. I breathe deeply, willing my heart to slow its thunderous beating. I close my eyes, but behind closed lids, a highlight reel begins to play: the missed answers, items not checked off on the perpetual to-do list, spilled milk on the floor of my kitchen, not moving quite fast enough and still missing details. Even if I run fast enough on the hamster wheel not to fall, will I ever escape it? It feels like drowning. Inadequacy crashes around my eyes and ears like a tsunami. I turn over onto my left side, adjust, then turn right again.

I wonder if I actually believe that one day, I won't feel this. I hope it's true. Perhaps by some power of osmosis, or the naturally acquired wisdom of age, liberation from imposter syndrome, from striving, from comparison verging on envy will one day just... And again, I drift off.

A few hours later, I'm awoken again. This time with an attitude of indignation. Is this all part of what medical school tactfully described as the process of "lifelong learning"? Of the continuous improvement that drives innovation? I huff, resentfully. Is this feeling supposed to be good, healthy, even? Some part of me can't help but wonder: When does the chase for some feeling of confidence, of comfort, transform from torturous to exciting? I flop onto my back, resigned.

After what might have been mere moments or many hours, something gentle settles over me. And the whisper of a question, from where I don't know, begins to form: Could I be loved without my flaws? More pressing still, could I love others without theirs? I look over at my husband, resting peacefully in the glow of the slowly brightening morning light. I think of my patients, the number of choices and uncontrollable circumstances that had to occur for us to meet in the hospital. How could I sustain a marriage, or decades of a medical career, without a personal understanding, passion, even love, of human fragility? What would remind us of our identical humanity, if not the unique weaknesses we share?

I remember all the hours, the sleepless nights spent desiring a mind that couldn't falter, and a body that could never grow old, weak or ill. I vow to spend my next sleepless night counting mistakes like sheep, with gratitude. •

Thought questions:
- Is it humanly possible to be as perfect as depicted in the author's nightmare?
- What are three memories that remind you of shared human fragility? How do these memories make you feel?
- What is something that you consider a personal flaw that has actually helped you or someone else?

Behind Closed Doors: Reimagining How Doctors Talk About Patients

•

Zachary Simpson

Before he stepped foot in my office, he had been marked.
"He's a difficult one," my boss warned me as he relayed this new client's backstory to me. I was working as a case manager at a community mental health center before starting medical school. My job entailed working with a diverse patient population, many of whom were experiencing homelessness, and linking them with community resources to help meet their basic needs. This new client had seen a litany of case managers before me and had a history of "non-compliance" with services, along with numerous documented missed calls and missed appointments. As he stepped out of my office, my boss paused and looked over his shoulder saying, "And by the way... he can get angry," before closing the door behind him.

At our first appointment, the energy changed as soon as this client stepped foot into the room. His clothes unwashed and hair unkempt, it was clear that he had been living on the streets. He angrily slammed my office door shut and began to yell; I rushed to grab a pen to jot down his requests, bristling as the list before me continued to grow and grow. When he had finished talking, I looked up and noticed him fuming in my direction. Without even realizing it, my body had tensed up, adopting an almost defensive posture at the onslaught of requests and demands. Seemingly everything in his life needed fixing, and we only had thirty minutes together. By the time he left my office, I found myself frustrated—both with him for not seemingly even giving me a chance and with myself for get riled up in the first place. Why had I been so prepared to be frustrated, so prepared to reflexively perceive the timbre of the conversation as a personal attack on me?

•

PREMEDICAL PERFECTION

From the moment I started medical school, I was sold on psychiatry. Psychiatry, to me, encompassed all that was thrilling about medicine—the detective work, the storytelling, and the human connection all wrapped into one delicious specialty. As I spent time rotating through different clinical environments, I couldn't help but feel aligned with the field itself, one driven by years of reshaping and revitalization, on the precipice of its future. I couldn't help but relate.

As of this writing, I am in my fourth year of medical school, currently in the process of interviewing for psychiatry residency and contemplating my own future. In this period of relative quiet, I have found myself with more time to reflect on the past three years of my training as I prepare for the next four. In my time between virtual interviews, slightly distanced from the rigid architecture that is medical school, complete with the continuous cycle of clerkships, grades, and evaluations, I am now able to more freely examine what these years have really meant to me and what I hope to carry with me into this next leg of my training. It is not lost in me that I have grown tremendously since I first started medical school, thanks in large part to the dedication of faculty and staff committed to training the next generation of physicians. Beyond that, though, I find myself contemplating the larger medical system—the one to which we are all to some extent complicit in shaping. How has this system shaped me (for better or for worse)?

Psychiatry as a field has not been without its struggles. As a specialty that relies heavily on history-taking and verbal communication with patients, language can make or break an interaction with a patient. These nuances of language are not unique to psychiatry, though. The physician-patient interaction at its core is storytelling, including both the stories patients tell us and the stories we hear. One of the biggest barriers to rectifying these often-disparate versions of the same story is a failure of providers to adequately acknowledge how the physician-patient interaction can be affected by the larger environment in which medicine is practiced, one where patient handoff can become a dicey game of telephone if we are not careful. This can manifest in the ways members of the health care team discuss patients when they are not around. Word choices that frame patients as "difficult," "time-consuming," "non-compliant," or "needy" fail to appreciate patients' complex histories with health care, especially when speaking about traditionally marginalized groups. Not only that, the language we use to discuss patients behind closed doors has the potential to prime other providers to interact with patients in ways that align with our own personal biases. Time constraints and frenetic pagers unfortunately sometimes reduce patients to buzzwords and first impressions, often to patients' detriment. Psychiatry has not been immune to these transgressions in language. In fact, it has often left the most damage.

The advent of the electronic medical record has made it easier for doctors to communicate about patients. The sharing of virtual patient information has the potential to help facilitate continuity of care, a convenient way to addend the ever-growing and often complicated medical histories of patients seeking care from a multitude of providers. Throughout patients' journeys through the health care system, through different providers, medical specialties, and hospital systems, they often get sidled with a multitude of labels, a shorthand to allow physicians to communicate about patients and their medical histories. These labels are often carried on and furthered through the sharing of medical records through different providers. These labels become, in some instances, not just part of patients' stories, but come to represent patients themselves. And here comes the rub—how difficult is it to *change* this story, to not only addend, but amend doctors' different interpretations and conceptions of patients' stories, documented and often cemented in this ever-expanding electronic diary of patients' health care journeys?

As a future health care professional, on the brink of starting residency training, it is imperative to acknowledge the history of trauma many people have faced—and continue to face—at the hands of well-intentioned health care providers. Nearing the beginning of my medical career, I want to commit to helping enact a culture shift, specifically around the way we talk about patients. It is in our patient's best interest—and our own—to set ourselves up for success before we even step foot in the room, framing our conversations around patient care in ways that lift patients up because how we talk about patients outside the exam room has the potential to affect the care they receive within the exam room. Patients deserve a chance to tell their own stories without being marked or branded beforehand with well-intentioned but sinister labels that end up telling their stories for them, poisoning the well before they're even seen.

•

Almost a year after we first met, this patient and I were sitting in my office at what would be our last appointment. In a month's time, I was starting medical school. I told him I was thinking about psychiatry, and he smiled. In our year working together, he had turned from a client I dreaded meeting to a client I looked forward to meeting. I realized that the "difficult" label he had unceremoniously been given before we met did not tell the whole story. He did. And as he opened up with me over our year working together and began telling me that story, I couldn't help but be humbled. We did not become instant friends. The work to build up trust was gradual, and at times, painstaking. I had to set my own self to the side, with all the preconceptions and gut reactions, in order to create space for the person in front of me. When he left my office for the last time, he thanked me. For what exactly, he didn't say, but I knew. He told his own story. And that had made all the difference. •

Thought questions:
- How have you seen labels detrimentally affect patient care?
- What have you noticed in your body when you encounter a "difficult" patient and what do you do with that sensation?
- Can describing patients as 'difficult' ever be useful? If so, when, where and how?
- Can you remember a 'difficult' patient? Imagine or practice with a friend how you would describe them to a colleague in a way that avoids creating bias?

The Journey

•

how doctors learned
to own their perfection

THE JOURNEY

I Was Not Her

•

Eve Makoff

Blunt cut hair, round glasses, skirt below the knee—she held herself the same way when she met patients and students. She was understated, deliberate, and gentle. I imagined that her heart beat at a measured pace, while mine raced. I was easily agitated by the commotion at the nursing station, or the news of an earthquake back home on a patient's silenced television. Or a patient's grief.

We were gathered outside the hospital room gripping index cards scribbled with lab values and diagnoses on our internal medicine rotation. Dr. Lyr was our attending physician. Inside the room, our sea of white coats formed a restless U. A dozen eyes peered down at the tiny woman under the sheets. Dr. Lyr pulled up a chair and sat eye-to-eye with our patient, warming an encounter that might have otherwise felt clinical and cold. Mrs. Laurel's veiny hand wrapped in her own, Dr. Lyr sat back and listened for as long as it took. There was no rushing past what the patient needed. And once the visit was over, Dr. Lyr helped us carefully craft our list of differential diagnoses. I wanted to be that calm, that dignified, that brilliant.

"I'm going to be a surgeon," I told her one day.

Her eyes crinkled, "No you're not. You're one of us. You'll see."

She was right. On my surgery rotation, I felt ill at ease. In the operating room, Dr. Foyer, his mustache bulging under the mask, berated Chief Resident Flowers for anything and nothing just to show life was going to be hard *if* she continued on this path. Through her glasses, I saw her eyelashes forming wet triangles. Holding the retractors, my chest ached. I increased the tension, trying to maintain a clear surgical field, wanting Dr. Flowers to succeed, but not wanting to follow in her wake. I knew I'd drown in those waters.

When I told Dr. Lyr I was considering California for internal medicine training, she said, "Remember, there are no earthquakes in Rhode Island." My heart swelled hearing that she thought I was worthy of staying nearby and working under her care. I, who wore bold prints and short skirts, who cried easily (and sometimes created personal drama), was deemed good enough to continue in the same halls as she? I felt too messy, too emotional, too *something*, to be worthy. It would be years before I understood I was.

THE PERFECT DOCTOR

•

Shortly after I entered practice as an attending physician, technology was inserted between doctor and patient. Instead of sitting by beds and looking in patients' eyes, we stared at computer screens to finish orders and notes. Under pressure, doctors were becoming more rushed and stressed out, with patient needs shrinking into the background. I thought back to Dr. Lyr and had the sense I was letting her, and myself, down. I didn't even have time to make the easy connections with patients that were my hallmark by that time. Now, everything was about evidence and efficiency. After acquiring the requisite medical knowledge, and harnessing my softer skills, instead of finally feeling good enough, I felt the opposite—like I was getting worse. I had a deep sense something had to change or I might break. And something did break.

In 2012, I had a non-aneurysmal subarachnoid hemorrhage. I spent nine days in the neurologic intensive care unit on pain medication and on watch for a stroke. At the time I was already contemplating a switch from internal medicine to palliative care so that I could slow down and focus on what really mattered to me, the relationship between a doctor and her patient. Although I eventually came back 100 percent physically, I was not ever the same person again when I returned to medicine.

Within months of my return to work, I had my first palliative care patient. She was in her thirties and had a chronic form of pancreatic cancer, less serious than adenocarcinoma. She received monthly intravenous infusions through a port catheter in her chest. She got admitted often to the hospital for infections, the price she paid for an in-dwelling line and a medication that was keeping her healthy. I was still fragile—weak, too thin from the bed rest that atrophied my muscles. I sat at her bedside in a mauve pleather chair. She was anxious, worried about her children, even though they were home safe with her doting husband.

"They need their mom. And I spend so much time here. It's got to be so hard on them, so confusing, you know?"

"I understand. I'm a mom, too," I said.

"Will I be okay?" she asked.

My eyes welled up. I couldn't help but think back to that moment in the emergency room when a CT scan confirmed I'd had a brain bleed, and when the doctor, my friend, had said I had "the good kind of bleed" but still had to go into the ICU. I thought back to my children's writhing little bodies as they climbed on my bed and got tangled in the wires attached to my chest and my limbs.

I took a breath and let the tears settle. I took her hand and told her what I knew about the truth of that moment. From then on, each time she came into the hospital, she asked for me. And each time I came and cared for her in the best way I could, attending to her worries, and answering her questions.

THE JOURNEY

I'd learned that it was okay to be emotional with my patients. Maybe better than okay, maybe essential. I also finally realized that I was good enough, or even just *good*—worthy of taking care of other people at their greatest time of need.

Although I never spoke to Dr. Lyr again, I finally understood what she saw in me all those years ago: a young doctor with a big heart who would one day know the power, the beauty, of deep feelings and vulnerability.

She didn't ask me to be her. I'd always been enough just being me. •

Thought questions:
- Is it okay to share emotions in medicine? With patients, with colleagues?
- How is sharing emotions at work beneficial and how can it be harmful?
- How can *not* sharing emotions in medicine be helpful or harmful?

THE PERFECT DOCTOR

My Mirage of Meaning

•

Audrey Nath

The cure for survivor's guilt? Perfection.

This story begins long before the white coat ceremony and taking the Hippocratic Oath. Long before standing on the front steps of my medical school to open that fateful envelope on Match Day. Long before the nights in the hospital with upper level residents and attendings, my first teacher was my brother. Initially, he was somewhat disappointed by my existence; he was four years old when I was born, and lamented, "When is she going to become a *real person*?"

But as the months and years passed, he was around to help me walk. And show me how to build landscapes out of Legos. One time, when I was three, he tried to teach me how to write, and I couldn't manage more than a few scribbles. He ran downstairs, disappointed.

But he kept on teaching me about the world around us. What I didn't realize at the time was that the biggest lesson of all that he would teach me wouldn't come until years after he was gone.

•

My brother died six months before I applied to medical school. We were weird kids. We had an expansive imaginary world full of named cats, one of which had its own pet gerbil. Our best memories were of the pixelated landscapes of 8-bit Nintendo games. We spent hot summer days watching Supermarket Sweep and eating Ovaltine out of the jar.

Nothing brought him back. But by God, maybe I could fix everything by being a raging success. Maybe it would all go away with some great publications during my PhD. Maybe I could make it all better by matching at Harvard for residency. And once I got there, by being the most efficient chief resident they had ever seen.

There was no hole in my soul, no regret or hopelessness that could not be filled with memorizing all the muscles, bones and blood vessels in the body. Every mechanism of every drug. Every life cycle of every bug. In short, I was desperately chasing perfection like a back-alley drunk looking

for the bottom of another bottle. It was my escape.
It was the solution, and cause, for all my problems.

•

What I couldn't shake was wondering why *I* was still here. What had I done to deserve to survive? I had a nagging feeling that I was still on this planet only due to dumb luck. Like there was no reason *at all* that it was him gone and not me. It must all be some cosmic joke. And it was during this time of grief and confusion that I dove headfirst into medical school.

Medical school is a wonderful place to go if you're running away from something. Like magic, your mind is filled with warfare amongst cells and biochemical cycles with no beginning and no end. Every page is filled with the molecular mechanisms of all human suffering, without actually having to think about what that *means*.

All of a sudden, I could no longer remember why I felt so lost; at any given moment, my mind was an endless loop of the last three facts I had read, repeating them in earnest, in an attempt to keep them from floating away. Even when going to the grocery store, I found that I had to write down my list of ingredients if it was a list of three items or more; any more just didn't fit.

And so, in this way, I floated along for months. Years. There were times that I didn't recognize myself in the mirror, but it didn't matter. Now, I had found a mirage of meaning: I had evidence by way of test results and board scores that could justify my existence.

The nagging thoughts of "Why am I here and why is he gone?" and "It doesn't make sense; he was the smart one and always had *all of the answers...*" could be balloons popped with decisive darts: I just *rocked* that shelf exam! I ate Step 1 for breakfast! Look at these first author publications! Finally, I had letters and numbers and percentiles and an H-index to assuage my survivor's guilt, and it was *intoxicating*.

•

It finally dawned on me one night, while on call, that I had no idea how I had ended up where I was. In a comedy of errors, I had a study to read but had notified the wrong tech. What was supposed to be a routine study in the early evening ended up turning into a multiple-hour goose chase to beg the right person to drive to the hospital in the middle of the night to perform the study. It wasn't a dramatic patient death or difficult family dynamic to navigate; it was this incredibly mundane turn of events which somehow released the question that I had buried for so long:

"What happened to my life, and what on *earth* am I doing here?"

I started retracing my steps, as if I had misplaced my reflex hammer an hour ago on a different floor and needed to find it. What led me to this fellowship? Why did I fight tooth and nail to get accepted to Harvard for residency? What fueled me to finish my PhD so quickly and prove that I was a raging success? And not just the one who...

...accidentally survived for *no reason.*

Oh, right. *That.*

That's why I'm here. That sinking, nagging feeling of guilt. The one I had tried to destroy with all the metrics of "perfection" that had been handed to me on a beautiful platter in medical training.

Guess it didn't work.

Whoops.

And so, in the ensuing weeks and months, I started to think about who my brother and I actually were. Not the stuff on paper, whether it be in an obituary or a résumé. What we were all about. What made us laugh. What were our dreams. I finally made the realization that he would've been my biggest supporter in me just being *me*. Not the artificial papier-mâché me, made of strips of diplomas and manuscripts and grants formed in my general shape, dipped in glue, covering up nothing but an empty balloon.

Slowly, I dipped my toes back into my core being. I started writing comedy. And performing comedy. And writing music. And focusing my medical mind on ripping apart cases of medical neglect of incarcerated people. I wasn't working on grants anymore; my days were filled with talking with public defenders and media appearances here and there, to advocate for the causes I believed in. It had absolutely nothing to do with my carefully curated, "perfect" academic trajectory and storyline that I had spent 14 years building. But by God, it felt *right*. I could see my brother nodding along with everything I was working on.

I eventually left full-time academics altogether, to give me more time and freedom to just, well, be me. My path now might not look like perfection. But it's so much more.

It's everything we *ever dreamed of.* •

Thought questions:
- What are your reasons for pursuing your life work?
- Have you ever questioned your motivations for your life pursuits? If so, what came of the question?
- What techniques for coping with tragedy most resonate with you?
- What role does medical education play in helping students find the path that is right for them? What about in helping students cope with tragedy?

THE JOURNEY

Learning to Attend

•

Kimberly Lee

I was not one of those kids who always wanted to be a doctor. I had no idea what I wanted to be. But I needed to get everything right.

When I was two, the grownups put me in a long white dress, gave me a basket of red rose petals, and sent me down a dark-blue-carpeted aisle. The bride would be following me, so I had to predict where she'd step and place each petal as precisely as possible. No way would I just scatter them profligately—what if I didn't have enough? And no way would I admit to anyone that I doubted my ability to do the job right. I just kept a tight grip on that basket.

And I kept a tight grip on the need to be right. I grew into the kid who could read anything by first grade and would readily correct teachers if they were wrong. I was annoyed when the organist used a different key for the hymns in church, and I cringed when the choir sang out of tune (turned out I had perfect pitch). When I practiced, I wanted to be sure I got all the notes right. When I wrote a paper, I wanted to be sure I got all the facts right. When I finally got an A minus in an upper-level history class as a college senior, I was shocked and offended.

By then I knew I'd be going to medical school. I had acquired information about medicine, as with everything else, by reading books. I told myself this career choice would keep me from "getting bored" and would also allow me to "help people." I was still hanging onto the need to know it all, convinced that others would need my hard-won expertise.

I loved med school. I took voluminous notes with a multi-colored "gunner pen" in the preclinical years and took pride in knowing more facts than the residents in the later years. I ended up in a highly competitive pediatric residency program, where I felt as though I finally fit in, but also feared I might never belong. I took it as a given that we, the doctors, were somehow distanced from the patients and their families—and, in retrospect, perhaps also from ourselves and from each other.

As interns, we learned that the upper-level residents referred to children with developmental delays, complex medical needs, and frequent hospital admissions as "members." Someone had apparently noticed that MRCP, which stands for Member of the Royal College of Physicians, also stood for what we then called "mental retardation/cerebral palsy." The "members" belonged to a reality disconnected from our own experience. Until we met these kids, whose names I still remember and whose faces I can still picture it: their various medical conditions were abstract bits of information—the "pearls" we collected for board exams. At that point, the pearls were more real than the people.

As residency went on, my career trajectory gradually shifted from primary care pediatrics to neonatology. Fetal/neonatal physiology and developmental processes fascinated me. So did the absence of uncertainty about patient compliance or inaccurate histories or anything else that went on in the larger world. NICU patients were captive and I could know everything about them.

But, of course, knowing things didn't necessarily translate into fixing things. The social determinants of health affecting many of our patients' moms were at least as daunting as the complex pathophysiology and multi-organ-system medical challenges of the babies themselves. Being able to figure out answers to exam questions didn't translate to being able to figure out what to do for an extremely preterm infant with complex congenital heart disease due to a genetic anomaly, too small for surgical repair but also too sick to grow—or a full-term baby with a birthweight over 13 pounds and associated birth injuries because his mom had uncontrolled diabetes and no medical care.

Neonatology can be like a multi-lane freeway, with traffic cutting in from all directions at varying speeds—and I didn't realize I needed practice driving. I didn't realize I needed to develop an inner sense of position, speed, and destination in relation to the external challenges. I remember crying once in the unit, exhausted, depleted, and probably angry. I thought the real problem was my own inadequacy and oversensitivity.

But once I finished fellowship, I could stuff all the uncertainty under an attending's long white coat with its empty pockets representing self-sufficiency. No need to carry anything around—the attending should know everything. I clung to my bits of knowledge like those long-ago rose petals.

So then what happened?

How did I, over a quarter-century, reach the vantage point of lofty insight from which I now write?

The interesting thing—or perhaps the predictable thing—is that there was no moment at which the clouds parted, the sun shone, and I grew up.

I never turned into the poised and remote and authoritative attending Sir William Osler described in his speech to medical students, *Aequanimitas* (Osler, 1914). I still catch myself struggling, more often than not, with frustration and resentment and not-enoughing. I'm still learning, so late in life, from the babies.

Neonatology does offer opportunities for contemplation, what educator and author Parker Palmer defines as "unveil(ing) the illusions that masquerade as reality... to see things as they are" (Parker, 1999). And the reality is that very little—besides the long white coat—separates me from my tiny incubated patients on life support, from their thrown-for-a-loop parents hoping for a quick fix, or from our trainees expecting to learn all the answers.

The information we need for board exams is different from the presence we need for our patients' families. And the delight that comes from getting things right on board exams is different from the delight of reconnecting with families at a NICU reunion—and finally realizing that "membership" may be a pearl of great price.

The reality is that uncertainty is woven into our lives, and delight is a pattern that emerges only in the process of learning. I'm learning that the basis for "what if" questions can change—from dread of expectations to delight in expectation.

I'm still learning to attend.

I'm learning that "attending" is not just a noun (a gerund)—something I am, a position I hold. "Attending" is also a verb (a present participle)—something I'm doing. An attending gets to pay attention and to be present with others. Not to know it all, not to fix it all, not to be the one in charge at all. But to try to see without "the lens of pathology" that encourages us to distance ourselves and "be taken up with abstraction" (Coles, 1989).

I'm learning that "perfect" is not only an adjective but a transitive verb—a part of speech that includes both actor and acted-upon. What if being perfected is a process? What if I am not so much self-sufficient actor as acted-upon in this process of becoming perfected, completed, made whole?

And what if all of us are, together, in process? What if, working together, we all create—and are created into—something greater than ourselves, by Someone greater than ourselves?

What if the empty pockets in the white coat make it possible to receive?

And what if receiving, in our emptiness, lets us slowly open, gradually let go, and freely scatter the petals we've been given? •

Thought questions:
- Will patients accept "the empty pockets in the white coat" of a doctor? Or, is there an expectation to know it all?
- What is an example from your life of being perfected or made whole?
- How has having an open mind served you in your practice or work? How do you remind yourself to keep an open mind?

THE PERFECT DOCTOR

The Arc of a Smile

•

Jazbeen Ahmad

She was a young woman who smiled and laughed frequently and easily. It was one of the ways she managed anxiety. When she was anxious, she used her positivity as a way to form human connection. The oldest of three, more than once in her life, she was summoned to use her happy demeanor to get a family member out of trouble. Once, she served as a moderator between school and a hot-tempered parent (her parent). She never honestly thought about how this skill set would play into being a physician. Creating quick bonds with others came somewhat easily to her and she assumed she would be able to communicate with patients and colleagues with ease. In medicine, relationships turned out to be more complicated.

Already at a disadvantage starting clinical rotations as a female South Asian American who went to medical school in the Caribbean, she wanted to stand out as intelligent, easy to teach, and punctual, if not always early. She was a person who smiled hello and asked how you were no matter how exhausted she was. However, she quickly picked up that her smile irritated those working long, grueling hours alongside her. In medicine, smiling people were assumed to be less focused and therefore not as intelligent.

Some time during her third year of medical school, she was standing in an operating room early on a Saturday morning. She had the opportunity to watch a zygomatic arch fracture repair. Before beginning, the surgeon cocked his head to the side and asked, "Do you already know everything I'm telling you? Why are you nodding?" She was crushed and embarrassed. She couldn't help but think that all her smiling while he was quizzing her in the physician's lounge had likely rubbed him the wrong way. To her and in her South Asian culture, nodding was a way of showing she was listening, *ah yes, interesting*. She never thought someone would be irritated by it. But there she was looking into the eyes of a clearly annoyed attending.

Medical school taught her: *Smile less. Refrain from appearing too eager, be well dressed but not too well dressed, and find a way to blend in and stand out. Study, know all the answers.*

She carried these lessons with her into an internal medicine residency. The pressure of being grilled and ridiculed in front of others went from 50 to 100 percent. The drama of alliances and friendships punctuated the stress of being a new doctor. She had no time to be sick, no time for herself or her family. She was learning, practicing, and failing. Her good nature was sucked out of her. Her smile faded as she dealt with the interworking of physician egos and the death that is all too great a reality in hospital medicine. She found no acceptable outlet to discuss failure or sadness.

"Haven't you had a bad outcome before?" Her attending gazed at her quizzically as she grappled with a patient's death. She had been working nights as a senior resident during a particularly awful year of influenza. She and her two interns responded to two rapid responses on the general medicine floor, while simultaneously managing a patient with impending respiratory failure in the intensive care unit. This shift ended with a cardiac arrest during shift change and ultimately a death. She cried at home until her heart hardened, and she became cold.

The genuine connections she had so easily made in the past faded, her family drifted further away, and her friendships melted as all her life became consumed by medicine. She dredged through, noticing that her voice now contained the somewhat snarky tone she had hated to hear in her attendings. Forever the optimist, the flame of which was now much dimmer, she continued to insist that medicine was her passion. She moved away from her friends and family to start a new job with a cold heart and PTSD from residency.

The loneliness was heavy in a new town but as she began to work, she began to feel appreciated and needed. Her patients and colleagues were kind and encouraging. She had her first child, a daughter, and her anxiety started to melt away. She began to smile again. She let the walls fall around her heart. She allowed herself to cry when she saw life pass before her eyes. She admitted when she didn't know all the answers. She didn't care if anyone noticed her flaws, and the strangest thing happened: they cried with her and supported her. They did not chastise her for having a heart. They thanked her when she worked endlessly to find answers.

Nearly 15 years later, she is a mother of three with a strong sense of self. She finally has a handle on what being a good physician means to her, which is far from what it meant to her attendings. This South Asian American good-natured-now-woman values listening to patients and colleagues and being thorough. She has learned that being brilliant has little to do with your outward appearance, whether it's smiling, perpetually solemn, fancy, or in wrinkled scrubs. She has found her perfect physician by being whole. •

Thought questions:
- Do doctors need to be hardened to do their job well?
- Is it okay for doctors to cry? If so, when and where is it okay?
- Who would you trust more: a happy doctor or a stoic doctor? Is demeanor relevant to skill?
- Where do you draw the line on doctors showing feeling? What makes it too much or too little?

THE PERFECT DOCTOR

Gift

•

Sheenie Ambardar

"Perfectionism is self-abuse of the highest order." I remember reading these words by American psychologist and author Anne Wilson Schaef on a colorful, random, internet meme many years ago. Because I've always been open to being influenced by serendipitous pieces of pop wisdom, I took the meme to heart, printed it out, and allowed it to marinate in the back of my mind. Little did I know that those words would become friendly companions on my own ten-year journey to self-kindness and self-love; a journey that has brought me to where I am today: an adequate, thoroughly good enough, human being and physician.

The competitive process of getting into medical school and then completing exacting medical training may tell us otherwise, but striving for "perfect" is indeed self-abusive and wholly unnecessary. Some of the happiest people I know accept themselves for who they are, speak lovingly to themselves despite their flaws, and do what they want, when they want. They move through the world with an easy confidence and a certain *joie de vivre*. Unburdened by excessive external pressures, they courageously follow the stirrings of their own hearts. Sadly, this way of being is one that the conformist, fastidious environment of medical training doesn't encourage and likely can't accommodate: it's just not the nature of the modern medical beast.

My own conflicted relationship with perfectionism began much before medical school, at the startlingly young age of five or six. That's when I remember thinking that I wasn't too fond of math and asked my parents why I needed to learn it. Without a pause they said: "Because when you're a surgeon and the patient is cut open on the operating table, you need to be able to count how many parts are inside." Their answer was funny; it would be even funnier if I hadn't taken their words so seriously. That's all it took to squelch my tiny, barely noticeable protest. Even at that age, I intuitively understood that being a good daughter, *the perfect daughter*, meant math, medicine, surgery, and most of all, making my parents happy at the expense of myself. Of course, I went on to become a math whiz in high school, all the while never really loving (or being particularly good at) math. And years later, I dutifully entered surgery residency, suffered through a miserable surgical intern year, and then thankfully came to my senses and switched to psychiatry.

Now, as a psychiatrist, psychotherapist, and coach, I truly enjoy seeing the lightbulb go on when I tell my most self-abnegating, self-critical patients: *"Perfectionism is the highest form of self-abuse."* They usually stop for a breath, taking in the profound meaning of these simple words.

"Dr. Ambardar, I've never heard that before."

"Dr. Ambardar, are you saying that I can still accomplish great things even if I don't harshly criticize myself?"

"Doc, I'm just worried that all this talk of self-love and self-compassion will make me weak and lazy."

No, no it won't. To have an internally felt sense that you are *adequate* no matter what you do or don't achieve, that you are *good enough* whether you love or hate math, is a magical soothing balm for depressed and anxious souls. It is a deceptively simple message that we should have all gotten in our childhoods. It is, I believe, the greatest psychological gift you can give yourself. •

Thought questions:
- Self-love is easier said than done. What are practices to help instill self-love and compassion?
- Can self-love itself be subject to perfectionism? i.e., "I am not perfect at loving myself." How can this be avoided?
- Is it possible to have *joie de vivre* and still push yourself to be the best doctor you can be?

… THE PERFECT DOCTOR

Signs And Symptoms: The Beginning—and Ending—of a Psychologist's Career

•

Melinda Ginne

In the early 1980s, I was in my mid-thirties, a never-married, commune-dwelling, curly-headed, Berkeley feminist. Having been raised by a seriously mentally ill mother who not only dominated my childhood with cruelty and unrepentant unpredictability, she had also taken up lodging in my head and was living there rent free. It was no surprise that I found my calling as a psychologist by the ripe-old age of sixteen.

It took fifteen years of education and training to become a licensed psychologist. En route, I worked my way through grad school with odd jobs—as a waitress in a diner, a night janitor at a mom-and-pop health-food store, a dog show specialty groomer. Somehow that stellar employment background landed me my first job as a psychologist by a major medical center in the San Francisco Bay Area. They hired me for my specialties in geriatrics (gero-psychology) and behavioral medicine, the branch of psychology dedicated to treating the psychological aspects of major medical illnesses. I'm sure the dog grooming must have tilted the scales in my favor.

After being on the job for six months, I went into the waiting room to greet my first patient of the day, whom I'll call Mrs. Leviston. She was in her early forties, dressed in beige stretch pants, a white cotton short-sleeved blouse, white ankle socks, and sneakers.

"Dr. Ginne, you have to help me with my fourteen-year-old son," she said as she sat in my office. She was clearly distraught. "He's so disrespectful to me and his father. He refuses to do his chores, and he's always arguing with his younger sister and brother. I'm at my wit's end—I don't know what to do with him!"

Hearing her story, I too, was at a complete loss. I had no idea what to do with him either. Beyond the basic child and adolescent theory classes taken in graduate school—which now seemed useless—I had no professional experience with children or adolescents. I had helped my best friend raise her son from the age of three until he was fifteen, but we basically treated him as a wild animal who we let sleep in the house, leaving him alone to raise himself, hoping he wouldn't kill us in our sleep. Somehow, I sensed that my experience wouldn't be of much comfort or support to Mrs. Leviston.

"Tell me a little more about yourself," I said, stalling. She told me that she was a homemaker, her husband a police officer. They lived in a nearby mostly working-class neighborhood.

"Honestly, Doctor, you have to help me. I've never seen a psychologist before, but I don't know where else to turn. My husband is ready to send our son to military school. I don't want that to happen!" She leaned in to whisper. "You know, Doctor, I don't like to spy on my son but... well, I do look through his drawers when I put his clothes away. And sometimes I listen in on his phone calls. But it's only because I'm worried about him, I'm sure you understand. Do you think I should ask our youth pastor to speak to him?"

Better him than me, I thought. "Does your son want that?"

"No, he doesn't want anything! He told me not to interfere."

I scrambled to recall what I'd learned about the rebellious teen years. But nothing I could think of seemed it would be of use. Furthermore, from what she said, I couldn't tell whether this was about the kid acting out or the mother being intrusive. While I knew nothing about adolescents, I did know something about mothers, especially intrusive mothers. Suddenly, I was struck with an idea.

"Mrs. Leviston, can I tell you a story?" She nodded. "I spent last summer in Mexico City, studying Spanish. Have you ever been to Mexico City?" She shook her head. "Well, the traffic there is absolutely crazy—cars pulling in and out of lanes, stopping in the middle of the street without warning, pedestrians ignoring lights and walking out in front of cars. It is total chaos. But I had to be able to get around town, so I took driving lessons. I remember something the teacher said: 'You cannot control the traffic or other people's actions. So the best thing you can do is to focus on the space in front of your vehicle. If you wish to avoid hitting another car or running over a pedestrian, you must focus your eyes on the few feet just beyond the hood.

"This turned out to be very good advice, Mrs. Leviston. Do you think you can do that with your son?"

She stared at me blankly.

"Keep your eyes on your own hood," I explained. "You know, have a restricted focus."

"Can I what?"

"Um, stay in your own lane."

Her eyes narrowed. She rubbed her lips together, brow furrowed, "Now I see," she said, with a nod, "Thank you, Doctor, you've made it so clear to me." There was a long pause, "I came here and told you about the trouble we are having with our son and that my husband wants to send him to military school. And you respond with some cockamamie story about focusing on my hood?"

Uh oh, this wasn't going well.

"'Focus on my hood, restrict my view, stay in my own lane,' what kind of nonsense is that? I'll tell you what it is. It's baloney, pure and simple hogwash!" She bent over in her seat, held her face in her hands, and moaned in anguish.

"I don't even know why I am talking to you," she said. Her face reddened, the veins in her neck bulged and pulsated. I gripped the arms of my chair.

"Why on earth am I wasting my time talking to you?" Standing up she declared, "You are such an idiot!"

With those words, she stormed out of my office. Instinctively, I ran out after her, spotting her at the end of the psychiatry department hallway.

"Wait!" I called out. "Please don't go, come back, Mrs. Leviston. I can fix this..." Doors opened. Several of the other psychologists stuck their heads out of their exam rooms. *Oh crap, how am I going to explain this at the Monday morning staff meeting?* Mrs. Leviston stood staring right into my eyes.

"Yep," she said. "That's right, a total idiot!"

She opened the exit door and, like The Road Runner in the cartoon, was gone in a flash. All that remained was a fleeting image of white ankle socks and sneakers.

I had no way to console myself, for she was absolutely right. I had been a total idiot, albeit an earnest and well-intentioned one. *Who was I to be helping other people figure out their lives when I couldn't even figure out my own.*

•

Thirty-five years after my encounter with Mrs. Leviston, I found myself nearing the end of my career. My work had been rewarding and successful—treating thousands of patients, collaborating with other medical specialists, teaching in graduate school, and mentoring graduate students.

Now in my sixties, I had a panel of over five hundred patients. I treated eighty people a week in a combination of individual, group, or phone appointments. Perhaps due to changes in the medical profession, perhaps due to my age, I often felt exhausted as well as discouraged.

I called the retirement center almost every month, "Can I go yet? Do I have enough credits to retire and get a pension?"

"Not yet, Dr. Ginne, you're almost there, but not quite yet. Just another year or two."

That seemed like a very long time. However, as weary as I was, I didn't feel quite done with my work. I needed something more—a sign that my work was complete.

One day I met a new patient, a woman in her eighties, who I'll call Mrs. Richardson.

"Dr. Ginne," she said, "I've been sad lately. Real sad. My sister died last year and I haven't been able to shake it. I miss her terribly. By the way, please call me Muriel."

She was stoic, though tears were forming in her eyes.

"I'm so sorry, Muriel, tell me about your sister. Did she live here in the Bay Area?"

"Oh yeah, Doc, we lived together, in a senior building right on the beach, in Alameda, the Gold Coast Gardens. Her name was Martha. Doc, we've been living together for the past fifty years."

"That's quite a long time. What did you and Martha do for a living?"

"I was a horticulturalist, Martha was a mystery writer."

"Did you and Martha grow up around here?"

"I did, I'm a third generation San Franciscan, Martha was raised in Chicago. She moved out here to earn a master's degree at UC Berkeley. We met in 1956 through mutual friends. I was twenty-six, she was twenty-nine."

Ah, now I knew what she meant as 'sister.'

"We courted for five years, then made it permanent when we moved in together. Only our closest friends knew about the nature of our relationship, we never told anyone else, no need really. But now that Martha is gone, I want people to know what we meant to each other, why she was so special to me, why it has been so hard for me to get back on my feet. Can you help me with this, Dr. G.?"

I thought of my schedule. For several years the providers and the management had been at odds with each other over access to care. Even my most medically ill patients were waiting months for a return visit. I would write emails to the chief of psychiatry asking for help with my caseload: "You can't ask me to tell a patient with four months to live that I'll see them in three months. I need to reduce my caseload so I can treat my patients in a more timely manner." The administration usually didn't reply to my emails, other than sending me a reminder to take a course on time management.

There was no way I could take on another patient. Even so, I found myself saying, "Sure, Muriel, I can help you. We'll find a way for you to honor Martha's memory and get back on your feet. Does that sound good to you?"

"That sounds real good, Doc. When can I come back?"

"I'll make an appointment for you to return in two months. In the meantime, I'll call you on the phone; we can check in that way. Is that okay?"

She nodded.

In our next session, Muriel told me more about Martha.

"She loved to read. She rarely left our room at Gold Coast Gardens. She didn't mind if I went out, she merely wanted to stay behind with her books. She loved poetry, especially women poets: Bronte, Dickinson, Maya Angelou, Anne Sexton, Adrienne Rich.

"Martha didn't care much for cooking, so she left that up to me. She was a skinny little thing, but she did love to eat. She especially liked when I fried up some pork chops or chicken thighs. She also liked my veggie lasagna. Oh, I do miss her, it isn't the same without her."

A few months later, Muriel reminisced about their life together. "Of course, nobody could be open about being a lesbian in the mid-1950s. Even dancing with a same-sex partner was illegal back then, but that didn't stop us. Instead of going to the bars, we formed a private lesbian social club where we had tea dances, BBQs, and glorious holiday parties. We were family, which meant so much to all of us who had been rejected by our own families. If anyone asked about the group, we said it was a poetry club. We loved our secret society where we could be open and honest about who we were and who we loved."

Before each meeting with Muriel, I thought deeply about how I could help her. I knew each session was important. After every visit I would say, "Would you like to make an appointment to come back to see me?" She always answered yes.

A year into our visits, she had progressed a lot. She attended a grief support group where she had been honest about her relationship to Martha, and no longer referred to her as her sister. She resumed some activities in her facility including field trips, a book club, and regular meals in the dining room. I referred her to an LGBT friendly visitor program and she felt that she had made a good friend in her visitor.

Two months later, at the end of our sixth visit, I asked the usual question, "Would you like to make an appointment to come back to see me?"

"Well, I think I would, but I have a question for you."

"What is it, Muriel, you can ask me anything."

"Well, you're such a nice lady. I did so enjoy our talk today. But there is one thing I'm wondering."

"Yes, please go ahead. I'm eager to hear what you have to say."

"Have we ever met before?"

Her question caught me off guard. I cleared my throat. I took a sip of water. I shuffled papers on my desk.

After all the hours I had poured into this case—the planning, the reflecting, the desire to be helpful—I was suddenly irrelevant. But not in a bad way, rather in a Buddhist way, as in the concept of having of "no-self." I had gone from being a total idiot to being somewhat enlightened.

It felt like a completed cycle, a full-circle moment. I wanted to hug her. She had shown me the sign I'd been waiting to see, the light at the end of the tunnel.

My work was done. •

Thought questions:
- Think of a time when a patient or someone did not like you? How did you cope? What would you have done differently?
- What would the *you* at the end of your career tell you early in your career?
- How do you find space for meaningful patient interactions during a busy clinical schedule? Is this up to each individual clinician, or up to leadership and the hospital systems to create time and space?

Lessons from Patients

•

lifelong learning
takes unexpected forms

Ricochet

·

Ajibike Lapite

Ava stood in front of the tombstone alone. The air smelled of rain from the night before and the grass was still damp. She regretted her choice to wear flip flops but had only half planned this visit to the cemetery. Her mother was at the park with Zoe and her husband was at work. It took just one offhand remark about a migraine for her mother to drive from Treme to the Bywater and insist that she take Zoe for the afternoon. Ava feigned resistance.

"Ava, who knows how much longer I have on this Earth! Are you going to deny me time with my only granddaughter?"

"Of course not," she answered.

She watched as her mother bustled about the kitchen in search of a clean sippy cup.

"What time is the appointment again, baby?"

Ava hesitated and then fumbled through the stack of opened letters on the kitchen table. Her mother found the blue sippy cup in the cupboard meant for bowls. She watched her mother frown as she glanced around the kitchen. She made no comment and Ava was grateful for her mother's restraint.

She found the appointment reminder from the children's hospital.

"It's early, Mama. Looks like it's at 9 a.m."

"Make sure that you get there on time. It's important."

"I know, Mama," she started.

She chose not to say that she had all but begged for Zoe's pediatrician to make the referral, that after the referral it took eight months for the appointment with the pediatric neurologist to be scheduled, that the "expedited" appointment for an evaluation by genetics came four months after the initial request, and that for the past four months that she had struggled to sleep.

"We won't be late."

Her mother poured equal parts water and apple juice into the cup and screwed on the lid.

"Can I go with you to the appointment? I don't want you to be alone."

"I'll call you right after. I promise."

Her mother nodded and grabbed Zoe's yellow jacket from the closet.

She passed the jacket over to Ava who pulled Zoe out of her playpen and into her arms. Her mother helped to slide Zoe's arms into the jacket and zipped her up. She kissed Zoe on the forehead before she passed her to her mother who put Zoe in the stroller.

She waved goodbye from the porch and then in a hurried fashion grabbed an umbrella and slipped on her flip flops. Later, she would say that she didn't remember driving over to St. Louis Cemetery #1, but that she must have. She would remember her shoes and the air and how she shuddered as she stood in front of the tombstone. The epitaph read Marie Laveau. She had been there twice before. The first time was nine years ago. She presented a bouquet of purple tulips and seven dimes and prayed for a husband. One week later, she met Andre.

The second time was one year ago when she presented a bottle of white rum and prayed for someone (just anyone) to listen to her concerns about Zoe. At first, she was frustrated that Zoe's 6-year-old check-up was with a new pediatrician at the practice. Later, she was grateful when Dr. Knight listened to her when she told her that Zoe was not who she was six months beforehand or even six months before that. She was even more grateful when the doctor ultimately recommended a neurology evaluation.

For years, Ava had tolerated when physicians shrugged and said that she should accept "Zoe time." Every child is different," one said. One printed out a copy of the Denver Developmental Milestones Chart. "See," he said "there is a range of quote unquote normal timelines for development. Zoe is consistently at the lower limit of normal. Her consistency is reassuring to me and I hope reassuring to you as well."

She was satisfied by that response when she sat beside her daughter in the clinic. Outside of that space, she was nervous. Her anxieties were quieted when Zoe spoke her first word at 16 months. It was "Mama."

•

Andre and Ava danced on their fresh-painted sage green porch after they heard her voice for the first time. Her voice was all the music they needed.

"She's going to be okay," Andre said.

She believed him until the music stopped. Zoe was just shy of her second birthday when she spoke for the last time.

"She's going to be okay," Andre said.

Ava laid her head against her husband's shoulder as she wept. She had burst with rage that surprised her when Zoe spilled a glass of apple juice all over the table. She had not noticed that Zoe's grasp had become less certain. She later noticed how unsteady Zoe had become.

"She's going to be okay," Andre said. She sighed in response. She scrubbed the dishes as Andre held Zoe in his arms. "Tell your mama that you're going to be okay, sweet girl," he said as he bounced Zoe. She wondered if his escape from the home to work helped him to unburden his worries. She wondered if she had not left the Times-Picayune if everything would feel less heavy.

"She's going to be okay," Andre said.

"Okay, but will we?"

He did not have an answer.

Her hand quivered as she etched three X's on the tombstone. She turned around three times as per the tradition. She presented the emerald bracelet she had found at the French Market and prayed for both an answer and a cure. At her feet were the offerings of others who sought healing from the long-deceased Queen of Voodoo. Ava knew that both her mother and her husband would be distraught by her visit and even more so by her belief in the practice. She had attended mass at St. David's ever since she was a schoolgirl. She attended Bible study. She prayed with intent. She believed in what she had been taught by her parents, but she was desperate. And she wasn't sure that her faith in Marie invalidated her faith in God. She was certain that her mother would not understand.

Her mother's faith in God was unshakeable. Her mother and her friends had prayed for Zoe before the time of her conception. When Ava crossed into the third trimester, they placed hands on her womb and prayed for a safe delivery. They prayed for Zoe's success. They prayed for her health. And when Zoe was diagnosed with autism, they prayed for a miracle.

Andre believed in God as much as anyone else, but as an engineer he spoke more often about his belief in science. There were moments when Ava felt as though he prioritized the ever-changing opinion of medical professionals over their own lived experiences. He believed that with therapy and time, all would be well.

"When should we try for a second one?" he would ask when Zoe had been put to bed.

She had deflected this question for years with various excuses. Most recently, she had shared that she needed the peace of mind of the genetics evaluation. She recognized that her "obsession" (as he called it) to understand what had happened to Zoe created space between them. On moments such as these, as she stood in front of the tombstone alone, that space felt like a chasm.

Ava left the cemetery and returned home. "Yes, Mama," she said when her mother asked her if the headache had resolved. They sat on the royal blue couch in the sitting room. Mama played with the remote, blitzing between the news and reality TV and ultimately settling on *I Love Lucy*.

"We used to watch this together when you were younger," Mama said.

Zoe's body was between Ava's legs. Ava had loosened Zoe's hair earlier and combed through it with a homemade aloe vera mixture. She parted her hair into six perfect sections. She twisted her hair into medium sized twist decorated with pink spheres. Zoe flapped her arms in excitement in the way that she had over the past four years. She stared up at her mother and smiled. Ava pulled her into her arms and kissed her forehead.

"I remember. I still watch it from time to time. It comes on when Zoe takes her nap."

Her mother kissed Zoe's forehead and squeezed Ava's hand.

"Tomorrow is going to be okay, baby. Give your worries to God. Everything is in His hands."

"I know. I know."

"You know, my whole prayer group has you in their prayers."

"I know. I know."

•

That night, Ava's mind was filled with all that she did not know. "Andre," she whispered as she placed her hand on his shoulder. He was asleep. She rolled over and grabbed her tablet and typed *Dr. Bourgeois—genetics* for the umpteenth time.

She poured through every word of his bio on the children's hospital website; she read his interview in the Times-Picayune; she watched his recorded talk from TEDxNew Orleans; she stumbled upon a number of abstracts that she did not quite understand; she found the announcement from about eight years prior when the children's hospital had hired Dr. Bourgeois.

"We are very proud to have one of the leading pediatric geneticists in the country here at Children's. Dr. Bourgeois and his team will expand the pediatrics genetics department as an important step to provide comprehensive pediatric care here in New Orleans," it read.

She closed her tablet and closed her eyes.

•

Ava pushed Zoe in her oversized stroller and checked into the appointment. They arrived early and waited just outside the front door until it was unlocked.

She scrawled "Zoe Landry" on the first line of the list on the clipboard. She pulled Zoe out of her stroller so that the nurse could take her height and weight. She held Zoe's hand as she took tentative steps from the scale to exam room #3.

"Dr. Bourgeois will see y'all soon," the nurse shared while taking Zoe's vital signs before she left the room. Zoe protested from the examination table and Ava stood up from the red chair and held her in her arms. She rocked her back and forth and then walked back over to the chair.

She sat on the chair with Zoe on her lap. "After this appointment, we'll get beignets, sweet girl," she said. Zoe flapped her arms as she did when she was excited. As they waited, Ava looked around the room. She noticed the hue of the paint on the walls—somewhere between tan and beige. She noticed the ophthalmoscope and otoscope were crooked on the wall. She looked down at Zoe, whose eyes were fixed on the episode of *Arthur* she pulled up on the tablet. She looked at the wall clock. It was 9:45 a.m. She pulled out her cell phone and texted her mother. *Still waiting on the doctor,* she wrote. *I will let you know everything after we wrap up.*

She heard a knock on a door which she answered with, "Come in."

"I'm Dr. Bourgeois," said the man who entered the room. He was dressed in a long white coat, a mint green long-sleeve dress shirt, and black slacks. "I have a few learners with me today who are very excited to meet Zoe as well."

"Okay," she said as five additional individuals entered the room. Two introduced themselves as medical students. One introduced herself as a pediatrics resident who was interested in a career in genetics. One introduced herself as an undergraduate who was in Dr. Bourgeois's lab. The last introduced himself as one of the genetic counselors.

"How old is Zoe?" Dr. Bourgeois asked.

"She's turning seven in a few weeks," Ava answered. She was surprised by the number of individuals in the room. She held Zoe closer.

"So, the first thing I notice," Dr. Bourgeois said as he walked toward Zoe to take a closer look "is that Zoe looks much younger than almost seven. What do y'all notice?" He stepped out of their line of view.

"Microcephaly," said the resident.

"Explain what that is for the students," he pressed.

"Oh, microcephaly means that her head is smaller than one would expect. The best way to be certain is to take a measuring tape to measure the head circumference and to compare it to the published standards for age." She gestured for one of the medical students to grab the measuring tape that she kept in her white coat pocket.

One took the tape and encircled Zoe's head. Ava made eye contact with her and she watched the student balk and then restart her measurement. She wondered if the student could sense her shock and her discomfort. She wondered if the appointment reminder had mentioned that the appointment would feel like a circus.

Each student was given an opportunity to ask questions about Zoe. From her uneventful delivery, to her hospital admission at 18 months for bronchiolitis, to her developmental milestones. Ava noticed that the resident glanced over at Dr. Bourgeois as she mentioned the time point for skill emergence. She also noticed the discomfort as she mentioned which of these skills had seemingly disappeared.

"A doctor a few years ago diagnosed Zoe with autism, but I didn't think that made sense. I know a number of folks with children with autism and none of them have ever noticed that their children were 'moving backwards.' I'm not sure the best way to describe it. I'm not sure if you know what I mean."

Dr. Bourgeois nodded. He looked at Ava briefly and then looked at his learners. "What is the term we use to describe this phenomenon?"

"Regression," the resident answered.

Regression. The word felt permanent in a way that worried Ava.

"So, what do we do for regression?" she asked as they pressed their stethoscopes on Zoe's body and examined every aspect of her body.

There was no immediate answer. The students glanced at one another.

"We like to identify the reason for regression first, which can help us think about next steps. The evaluation by neurology helps to rule out a number of things on the short list, which leaves genetic disorders as a potential explanation. I have no reason to believe that Ava has autism," Dr. Bourgeois started.

He said a number of things as the medical students shifted their balance from one foot to the other. The bravest of the group sat on the examination table. Ava heard the following fragments:

"The genetic studies sent by our neurology colleagues have returned."

"We have a genetic answer for the changes that have been concerning to your family."

"Zoe has Rett syndrome."

"De novo mutation."

"No cure."

Ava was not aware that she had started to cry until the genetic counselor passed her a green box of Kleenex. She grabbed the box and dabbed her eyes. She locked eyes with the medical student who took the head circumference. She noticed that the student had become tearful.

Rett syndrome: an answer. A diagnosis. Ava had hoped that a diagnosis would undo the years of questions and concerns and the shock she had felt when Zoe's capabilities (speech and dexterity) disappeared. She had hoped that a diagnosis would relieve her of the guilt that had become oppressive. She had hoped that the diagnosis would make clear to her husband that she had not been worried without reason. She had hoped that a diagnosis would mend the hurt she felt when she and Andre argued over whether this regression would be permanent.

Diagnoses at times can give rise to answers and hope and peace. Sometimes these diagnoses are destructive. Sometimes these diagnoses are twofold: answer and question alike.

"It was nice to meet you and Zoe. Let us know if you need anything," Dr. Bourgeois said before he left the room. The pack followed. He had not asked her if she had questions. She was not certain if she even had any.

•

She placed Zoe in the stroller. She leaned against the examination table as she called her mother.

"Baby, are you still waiting for that doctor? It's 10:00 a.m.! Do I need to come up there and tell them to be punctual?"

She opened her mouth to respond and found not words but sobs.
"Baby, what's wrong?"
"Baby, are you okay?"
"Baby, what did they say?"

•

She found three words that she repeated over and over again: "I don't know. I don't know. I don't know." •

Thought questions:
- How could Dr. Bourgeois have made this interaction less confusing and tragic for Ava?
- How can we both train students and residents in rare diseases and avoid patient's feeling like they are at the center of a circus?
- What touched you the most about Ava's story?

THE PERFECT DOCTOR

High Wire History

•

Melani Zuckerman

I sat in his shared hospital room, the curtain pulled halfway closed for a touch of privacy on the swarming oncology floor. I glanced at the clock, checking that I was still on target to complete my interview in the fifteen allotted minutes. Taking a deep, trepidatious inhale, I plunged headlong into the first-year students' most feared interaction: The Social History. This is the high wire portion of patient intake for the new medical student, and it is mined with potentially explosive situations at every corner. Armed with only a few defensive techniques and phrases, I balanced on that high wire, only to find that beneath my feet the net of protection was about to fail me in a visceral way. With deep hope and a generous sprinkle of naïveté, I proceeded.

"When was the last time you used alcohol?"

"Excuse me?"

"Sir, I was just inquiring about your substance use. When was the last time you consumed alcohol?"

"Why would you say that—assume that I drank? I've never had alcohol in my life!"

I immediately felt a cottonmouth sensation as my face flushed in a way that was palpable to me even without a mirror. The pen that I was clutching began to slide through my fingers; a cool clamminess dampened my composure as my nerves revealed themselves. I ran my hands over the bright white of my coat—not one month old, still starchy with idealism—stopping as my fingernails reached its end at my hips. As I searched my memory bank for some prerecorded escape hatch, I realized that the high wire on which I was ever so gingerly progressing was vibrating too intensely. Searching for the net beneath me, I found only gaping holes.

"Oh, I'm sorry sir, I had learned that this was a way to normalize alcohol use."

"Well, I wouldn't do that. I'm a nice guy, but someone else could get really offended!" His white eyebrows furrowed, and my attention directed to his pained expression. He sat up, revealing a bony frame and tubing draping over his arm.

"Everyone always just thinks I'm some big drinker. They see a thin guy in the hospital and just assume the worst. My dad was an alcoholic and I never touched the stuff after he died."

I had meticulously memorized every scenario outlined in the "Guide to the Social History" handed to me the week prior. I knew the delicate physician dance that gently prodded necessary items of personal information regarding sexual habits, substance use, intimate partner issues and a plethora of other necessary tidbits. I thought I knew how to implement the cardinal rule of non-judgement, as well. Despite my careful memorization of all these stopgap measures, I had managed to wreck this interaction with my failure to appear objective. I had become a medical student with a moral agenda, or at least that was what this patient saw. I was at a loss for words. I abruptly ended the interview with a heady feeling of incompetence and took a deep cleansing breath as I bolted out of the room.

In my attempt to normalize, I had ostracized. In trying to comfort and ease, I had offended and alienated. I headed home, thinking about all the ways I fell off my highwire and slipped through my safety net.

I returned home that night and took off the leather dress shoes that I was still breaking in. While nursing my blisters, I attempted to direct my attention to my histology course: *cuboidal, striated, intercalated, fimbriae, granuloma... why was he so upset with me... type III collagen, eosinophils... How would I say that better? Should I ask my preceptor?* I found myself unable to remain attentive to my exam that week. *How can I be a good doctor in a world where words hold so much baggage?*

After hours of struggling to balance my worries with my studies, I decided to shoot a text to my fourth-year preceptor in search of some more seasoned advice—something of a post-interview tradition for me at this point.

"Hey, I was just wondering what I could have done differently with that patient. I tried to say what we had learned in class. Did I say something wrong or was it an odd reaction from him?"

She replied with twelve words, which I later inscribed on a Post-It Note and affixed to my laptop: "There is no way to always be right. Don't worry about it."

•

While in clinical years, it is standard of care for medical students to be "pimped" by their attendings or residents. It was a new experience to be criticized by a patient, even more so in my first year. It has remained a flashbulb memory that I have somehow retained, despite most of my brain being inundated with the curricular firehose of medical school. However, the impression of that memory has softened and transformed from one that initially stung and ached to one that has formed healthy protective scar tissue.

Throughout the months that followed my preceptor's twelve-word response, I came to appreciate the inherent truth in the words stuck to my silver laptop. At the root of medicine is the absolute humanity, and therefore, fallibility of all interactions. I have learned that my white coat pocket is simply not deep enough to hold every permutation of patient encounter with the best way to conduct each interview cataloged for a quick glance between rounds. Not every high wire act needs a safety net that works—sometimes we are simply bound to fall through a hole. Interactions can be loaded weapons, and even as we try to use them as salves, or as magic, we do not always control their wild trajectory. Words carry different baggage to different ears.

I have since made peace with this basic fact. In my quest to be a perfect physician that never fails to use the ideal word, I will always come up short. I will never be able to phrase or state myself in a completely benign way. My own humanity, and my own beating heart will always inherently limit me. I can only do my best to learn and grow and reconfigure my approach through the years and decades to follow. Stagnancy can never be the plan, and my approach must evolve as my career moves forward. Occasional failure is all but assured, but this is an outcome that I must learn to embrace. That will not make me an inferior physician—it will make me a human one. •

Thought questions:
- Recall a time when you have been called out for your use of words despite best intentions. What did you do to correct the situation? What would you do differently next time?
- Can self-acceptance and perfectionism coexist?
- This story exemplifies how perfectionism can get in the way of learning and how the mental loop of failure can sabotage even the most capable brain. What else would you say to a friend or student or mentee who came to you after a similar patient interaction? Could you say the same thing to yourself?

LESSONS FROM PATIENTS

The Birth Plan

•

Andrea Eisenberg

I look up at the flashing monitor and scan for which little box is my patient. I've been sitting in the labor and delivery doctor's lounge for so long now that I have a collection of empty yogurt and fruit containers, a half-eaten salad, some cold coffee, and crumbs from my "chaos" cookie sitting next to me. Squinting to find my patient, room 3907, I finally get up to make sure I'm looking at the right labor strip. Not meaning to, I sigh loudly. The other obstetrician in the room looks up, "Everything okay?"

"Yes, just a long, slow labor for my patient."

I've been at the hospital twelve hours now, my patient twice as long. My time has been spent calling patients with lab results, rounding on those in the hospital, and intermittently checking on my patients in labor. She, on the other hand, has been pacing by her bed, sitting on a giant ball, and laying down in various positions. She came to the hospital yesterday after her water broke and had no contractions for several hours. Her original birth plan had been dashed hours ago when we agreed her labor needed to be augmented.

I remember discussing her birthing plan in the office a couple of weeks ago. She looked back and forth from her phone to me, reading off the list she had compiled, as if labor and birth could be planned to the T.

"I want a natural birth, skin to skin with my baby immediately after the birth, delayed cord clamping, no episiotomy, my husband to cut the cord..." She paused for a moment and then added "I think I want a doula there, this is my first baby..." she trails off. She looks at me expectantly. She knows I know it's her first baby. I can't tell if she is readying herself for battle and needing to justify her birth plan. Or perhaps she is reciting a plan that *she* thinks she should follow. Or she wants me to reassure her that her delivery will be all she hopes it will be.

"Tell me more about what you mean by a natural birth," I invite her.

Pregnancy and birthing are natural processes, after all. They are not illnesses or diseases that need to be cured. But obstetrics is a balancing act of caring for two patients at once—two patients who are intimately attached; one who has a voice, one who doesn't; one who can make decisions, one who can't; one who is independent to make choices, one who is dependent on the other. There are times though, one's needs must take priority, even if it's at the expense of the other.

This is the art of medicine—muddling through the gray areas of pregnancy and delivery when they don't go as planned. Sometimes, within this gray area, I am plagued by uncertainty and my limitations in knowing what would make the best outcome for both mother and baby. Overriding all this is the discomfort in potentially disappointing my patient by not giving her the dream delivery she desires.

Nature isn't perfect and can throw a loop in anyone's plans.

Sometimes babies are breech, or too small or too big, or have anomalies or defects. And other times the patient has health issues, like high blood pressure, diabetes, colitis, or kidney disease. We as physicians are trained to manage these issues and hopefully have a good outcome with a healthy baby and mother. However, it may dictate interventions that take away from a "perfect" delivery. There are times these issues come up suddenly, like a patient bleeding heavily from a placental abruption. Or are more insidious, when a baby just isn't fitting through the birth canal despite the patient pushing for hours and hours. For this reason, I try to encourage thinking of birth plans as not set in stone, but rather a guide that may need alterations along the way.

One by one, we went through her list, me mostly nodding as she talked.

She ended with an emphatic "I want no pain medication for sure!"

Once she was finished, I responded, "Since this is your first baby, it can be difficult to know what to expect. You may come into the hospital already completely dilated and ready to push or you may have a two-day labor. So, we may need to play things by ear. Let's talk a little about those scenarios."

But how do you explain the fatigue of labor, the relentless pain of contractions, the potential of hours of pushing for a typical first-time mom? How can anyone anticipate how they will react to labor and birthing? How do you know what you don't know?

When I was in labor, it didn't feel like I thought it would at all, even though I had seen and helped so many women labor. I pictured myself calm and collected, so calm that I would just labor at home, never make it to the hospital, and deliver in my bathtub instead. Ha! In reality, my first child was breech and I ended up having a C-section. With my second, my contractions came so quickly, I barely had a moment to recoup and get myself ready for the next. In the hospital, I stood beside my bed, white knuckled, hanging onto the rail, breathing to survive. I was never planning to get an epidural—my sister and sister-in-law never did, *I should be able to handle it too*, I thought. But there I was, in the throes of labor, trying to sit still as the anesthesiologist poked at my back. Each contraction felt like a wave throwing me into a craggy shore. How the heck was I supposed to sit still? In the fog of labor, I can't even remember asking for the epidural.

I stop my ruminations and look at my watch. *Five more minutes and I will go back into my patient's room.* And I sit again. *She's not going to be happy if she isn't dilated more.* But I'm concerned that the baby hasn't descended into her birth canal nearly the entire time she has been in labor. I'm concerned that she may get infected the longer her water is broken. I'm concerned the baby isn't fitting correctly in her pelvis.

I also know her birth plan has completely derailed. Here we are, twenty-four hours into her labor and she has barely made any progress. I'm dreading walking into her room again and seeing her tired face, her limp hair, her contorted body trying to manage the pain. And her disappointment.

I look at my watch again. It's only been two minutes.

Despite hundreds and hundreds—probably thousands—of beautiful, happy, "thankful for all you did" deliveries, I was haunted by those that didn't go as planned, had an unexpected complication, weren't the "perfect" birth. Like a slideshow, they sift through my brain.

The time I had to remove a patient's uterus right after I delivered her baby because the placenta had grown into the uterine wall. She bled and bled and the only way to save her was to do a hysterectomy. I looked over the blue drape at my patient and her husband as they held their baby. I tried to sound calm as I urgently spoke. "I'm sorry, but your placenta grew into your uterus and I have to remove your uterus. I can't stop the bleeding any other way." Her husband, without missing a beat, said, "Do what you have to, Doctor, just save my wife."

Or the time a patient broke her water at 22 weeks of pregnancy. She started contracting and there was nothing I could do to stop her labor. She cried and sobbed and moaned. "I can't kill my baby," she repeated over and over again. "I can't push." And so for hours she laid in bed with her baby half in her womb, half out. Her premature baby died within minutes of being delivered.

Or the patient who had pushed for hours. The baby was wedged deep in her pelvis, but wasn't fitting through the birth canal. She needed a C-section for her 10-plus pound baby during which her uterine incision extended into tearing her cervix. I had to call in for extra hands to help with visualizing and repairing her torn cervix.

Or the time my patient had such a severe headache along with severely high blood pressure that I had to induce her when her baby was two months premature. Despite my explanation of the concerns of her having a seizure or stroke, or even possibly dying, she wouldn't relent to the induction until she couldn't cope with the headache anymore.

Or the patient that, at her 20-week anatomy ultrasound, was found to have a baby with severe anomalies. Her baby would die, possibly while still growing in her womb, possibly after delivery where it would never cry or take a breath. I had to help her decide to continue or terminate the pregnancy, both of us knowing either decision would be a difficult road.

•

THE PERFECT DOCTOR

I finally get up and walk to her room. It's dark now and hard to make out her features in the shadows of the room. Her husband sits up from his perch on the couch, hair disheveled, blanket falling to the floor. He stretches and yawns. "So, what do you think Doc? We going to have this baby soon?" he asks.

I sit on the edge of her bed and ask, "Are you feeling the contractions at all? Any pressure?"

"Not really."

"Let me examine you since it has been a few hours and see where you are at."

As I touch her, her skin feels too hot. I turn to the nurse. "Can you take her temperature, please?"

Her cervical exam is unchanged and her baby's head feels like a conehead, trying to reshape to fit through the birth canal. The nurse tells me the patient's temperature—she now has a fever. And as I go to wash my hands, I can hear the baby's heart rate drop briefly.

I sit back down on the bed and run through what I'm thinking: my concerns about her obstructed labor, her fever, her baby. I discuss the options going forward. I look at my patient and see her fatigue, her frustration, her fear. I take her hand. "We need to make some decisions." •

Thought questions:
- What do you imagine the narrator of the story said next? How do you think the patient reacted?
- Is there a right and a wrong way to prepare a patient for the unexpected? What techniques do you think are most successful?
- Are patient's entitled to health care their way? If so, to what extent? Where can and should providers draw the line?

Paradox

Soma Sengupta

Can you cure my brain cancer?
I look into the eyes of my patient
A young man, with his life ahead of him
To be cut short by glioblastoma.
I evade the answer, he knows the answer,
Why is he asking me, what he knows?
Becoming a doctor, to make patients
Better, better for what and by what,
Asking myself, as the pager goes off
Again, and again, eating away at
Time—until I forget my own space
And I circle back to the question,
An imperfect answer to the question.
"We need to wait for your molecular
Markers, these are important..."
My voice fades away, he looks at me,
"I need to find that perfect doctor,
Who will tell me what I need to hear."
I wish him luck, and think, and think again,
There is no cure, and there is no perfection. •

Thought questions:
- How would you feel, faced with this question from a patient with an incurable type of cancer?
- How would you answer this question?
- Who is the perfect doctor that this patient seeks? What qualities do they posess? Do they exist?

The Redeemer

•

Jeffrey Millstein

I'm pretty certain it was Conrad who finally taught me to hear what patients were trying to tell me. I had taken plenty of patient "histories" through the years, but with Conrad there was no taking. You had to hear it the way he wanted to tell it. Period.

Conrad and I met years ago, back when I had a tendency to become slightly nauseous and clammy when I saw certain names on my schedule. Talkers. The ones who hijacked visits with their lists and chaotic soliloquies that seemed like they would never end. The tellers of tangential tales designed to keep me from important things, like diabetes management, bedside lectures on the dangers of smoking and taking medicine as instructed, cancer screening and the like. These patients made me step in like a referee, blow my whistle and take control of whatever time we had left with one of my stockpile of interruptions.

"Okay," I would say. "That's a very interesting story and I wish I could hear more, but we've got some serious work to do here."

"I'm going to stop you now, because we only have ten more minutes and a lot of things to go over."

I would joke with my staff and say, "If so-and-so is on the schedule, don't add anyone else. Visits with him should count as a full day's work!"

Conrad was a new patient who just happened to have the appointment right after so-and-so.

He sat wedged in next to the exam room desk in his electric scooter. Tangled oxygen tubing ran from a hissing tank in the front hanging basket to his nose without an inch to spare.

Conrad would have stood well over six feet if his legs would support him. He was in his early forties then, sporting a vintage Philadelphia Eagles jersey over his husky frame and espresso brown skin. His big grin was a perfect match to a deep, resonant baritone.

"Hey Doc! Conrad. Boy am I glad to see you," he said, beating me to the punch. As I introduced myself and we shook hands, I had already concluded that "glad to see you" meant he was about to unfurl a scroll brimming with complaints that were bound to further thwart my morning schedule.

We still used paper charts back then, and all I had to work with was the medical assistant's set of vitals, and "new patient" written under reason for visit.

"So what brings you in today, Conrad?" I was still using the all-business opening.

"Man," he let out a deep sigh. "I really need a good doctor."

"Okay, great. Tell me about your medical problems."

"How much time you got?" he replied with a snicker. Or maybe I just imagined the snicker while in the grip of the angry surge this comment always generated in me. I redirected.

"Maybe we can start by going over your medications?"

"We'll get to that," he said. "I've got my list in here somewhere." He pointed to a plastic convenience store bag stuffed with papers, envelopes and a pack of cigarettes. "See, I just moved in with my sister, 'cause I couldn't keep up my house no more. Since I got shot and all."

Conrad started to tell me about the fight he had in his old neighborhood a few years ago when a gunshot wound to the spine left him with only one fully functioning upper extremity and almost no leg strength. As he began to tell me the details of that fateful night, I felt a dreadful need to plot my exit strategy. At his soonest pause, I interjected like a predatory cat.

"Conrad, this is a very interesting story, b—"

"I'm glad you think so," he broke in with equal acuity and went on until I made my next move.

"Listen," I said, turning the volume up a couple of notches, "We haven't gotten to any of my—"

"Doc, I know you ain't got all day for me. There's just some stuff you got to know. We'll get to your stuff. Just hear me out for a few more minutes."

Conrad was beating me at my own game.

I sat with teeth clenched while Conrad told me the rest of his story. He went on about how he hadn't been able to work for years, and how difficult it had been to seek disability benefits and reliable health insurance coverage. Specialists kept adding on medications for diabetes and hypertension that were not covered by his meager prescription plan, which always led him down a gauntlet of misinformed doctor's office personnel to seek a solution. With no tactful escape plan, I began to listen as Conrad continued his hardship tale. Maneuvering away from the computer desk, I leaned back in my chair and did something strange and unfamiliar: I surrendered to his narrative.

All told, the visit took about forty minutes—ten beyond the allotted thirty for a new patient. In fact, if I hadn't pushed back and tried to force my agenda on Conrad at the beginning of the visit, we may have even finished on time. We got through most of his history, a very brief physical examination, and arranged for a follow up in a few weeks.

It took me a while to comprehend what really happened during that first visit with Conrad. All I knew right afterward, was that I felt less stressed than usual through the rest of my patient visits that day. At first, I thought that was simply because I was relieved to have finished up without being way behind schedule. The truth, I now see, was much more profound.

Conrad was much cleverer than he seemed. I came to learn that he hatched his caper years before we met, took his time rehearsing, finally working up the nerve to execute it. He was ready for the interruptions, the speeches, the re-directs, the over-talk. He was a student of the doctor-patient power dynamic, and approached it like a judo master, throwing me off balance with his own evasive conversational tactics. And I wasn't the first doctor he tried it out on, but recently he told me I was the first one who he came back to see a second time. And then a third. And then for the rest of the 20 years he had left before he died this week.

At his second visit, Conrad and I fist bumped, and I started with, "Hey Conrad, good to see you. What's at the top of your agenda today?" I thought he might think I was mocking him, but he must have seen the sincerity in my eyes. He simply said that he wanted to review his medications and make sure he was up to date on diabetes testing. He cared about his health, and just needed me to know him, and feel assured that I cared to listen.

I occasionally wonder if something more than medical need brought Conrad to me. There is enough mystery in the world to poke at my curiosity about forces which operate in some incomprehensible space. I'll never know. But something changed in me that day, like a rewiring. I was no longer in such a hurry to launch into my agenda. I actually enjoyed listening to patients and, even better, I liked how they seemed so grateful that I had. Sometimes I would even get a "Thank you for listening," or "I feel better just telling you what happened," as if they expected the same old hum drum holiday gift and were delighted to unwrap a luxurious surprise.

I admit that some patients still push my buttons. When triggered, I've learned to conjure a mental image of Conrad. Like a compass, he offers wayfinding with his admonishing grimace, and then his subtle smile when I reorient the visit in a more positive and compassionate direction. Thanks to Conrad I'm no longer trying to be the master of the exam-room universe. Instead, I am a receiver of stories. And it has made all the difference. •

Thought questions:
- If you work in health care or a service industry, describe a patient or client who has taught you something. How did that change your practice?
- Think of a doctor who you have witnessed connect with a patient. What qualities did they demonstrate and what techniques did they employ?
- Describe the ideal power dynamic between doctor and patient. Should the doctor be in charge? Should the patient lead the way? Should they strike a balance? If so, how?
- How should a doctor or patient make it known that their needs and responsibilities are not being met in a doctor's visit?
- Does the medical system need to adjust to make more time for patient's complex needs? If so, how and why?

LESSONS FROM PATIENTS

Octavian Was His Favorite Emperor

•

Anna Böhler

Not even a year ago, I had a very good friend, a friend with whom you don't have to mince matters. He was a tall man and his posture was always a little bit bent forward. It was as if he had to duck down to observe the world attentively with his soft brown eyes. He was exceptionally literate and well aware of that fact. In contrast to others, however, he was a quite humble guy. He loved to wear Scottish scarfs. He had at least a full dozen of them, and he collected gemstones and ancient coins. Let's call my friend O, because Octavian, the first Augustus, was his favorite Roman emperor. He always wanted to give this name to his child (at least as a second name, as he recognized the difficulty of convincing a potential future mother of that choice).

But my friend O had a condition. Since he was 12 years of age, he suffered from ulcerative colitis. His progression was severe. He had multiple hospital admissions, with doctors wondering many times how he could still be alive with hemoglobin that low. From his childhood on, he had various doctors taking care of him. They tried multiple different therapies, which quickly led into the wide array of off-label-study-based-approaches. Despite the efforts, he had discomfort almost every day and nothing really improved his condition.

He was diagnosed with colon cancer when he was 26 years of age. He got a colectomy and had a protective stoma for weeks. O was scattered and suffered a lot during that time, but his surgeon calmed him down with down-to-earth arguments. "Get the colon out and everything will be good!" was his slogan. O repeated it many times when we talked about that topic. Indeed, O had problems in the beginning, but the stoma got relocated and O soon came along with his new intestine pretty well.

Alas, it was just a brief respite, since only a few months later an MRI showed suspicious lesions scattered in his liver. He got diagnosed with a new, second tumor of a different origin—inoperable. O had to change his doctors now and had to consult the oncology department of the university clinic. From there on he went through an even worse cycle of chemotherapies, infections, frustratingly ambiguous radiological results, and a myriad of suffering and pain ensued.

As a friend, I felt completely helpless. Before, we never had problems with talking, nor quarreling. But as O's conditions got worse, my tongue became so heavy. Sometimes, my head felt like a parched desert of words. I knew I couldn't do anything to help him with the very big questions. Instead, I tried to interpret the blood tests and radiological results with him and checked on the information sheets of all his drugs. Surprisingly, he himself also wanted to talk about these "small" things over and over again. Probably to distract himself or to hold onto the feeling of being in charge, of maintaining control over what happened to his body.

He had great trust in his doctors. But sadly at this point at the clinic, he didn't get what he needed. No one there, except for some, mostly female, interns and nursing staff, would talk to him the way he expected and wanted.

My friend O died at 28 years of age. He fell asleep after receiving a last dose of morphine late at night in a small hospice where his mother brought him two days before. The last time we talked on the phone, a week before he died, he didn't share his anxieties about the illness. He did not even talk much about his severe pain. He just vented for over one hour about the lack of basic human attention that he suffered in that hospital and the smug medical staff. He was suffering, but he was at home and did not want to return to the university clinic. O was a very brave character, but the prospect of getting wrapped in that tense atmosphere again, where communication was reduced to a very minimum as if there was something sleazy about it shook him with such great fear.

O was a great admirer of old German literature. There is the famous story of the knight Parsifal that I think about a lot. Parsifal's destiny was to become king of the Holy Grail, but he got kicked out of the Castle of the Grail in disgrace during his first visit there because he missed a simple thing, a small question. He did not ask the old king, who sat silent and sick on his throne, what was going on because he felt spending more words than necessary would be a sign of weakness. As a result, he then had to wander around for years and years to find the Holy Grail again.

If there is one thing that I learned from O's terrible story, it is this: A lack of shared words can cause and aggravate illness. Of course, uncertainty is omnipresent in medicine, but it should be addressed. Naming uncertainty is not a sign of weakness. In fact, asking and listening can rarely be wrong. I think my friend O received the best medical treatment possible. But nevertheless, he suffered so much from these immaterial things, from this lack of words.

I always thought that to work as a doctor, you must be excellent in every aspect technically, socially, and empathetically. This is a very high measuring stick that frightened me often, probably because in reality it is a state too exceptional to be reached.

It may be expected that a doctor always helps and knows the way. But a doctor is also just a human being and, like everyone else, he or she will rarely do everything right. At the very least, we can try being patient and open with our patients. Therefore, Parsifal's attempt and failure to gain the Holy Grail seems to be a good allegory to keep in mind. •

Thought questions:
- Have you, or a family member, or a friend had an experience in which you or they felt unheard by doctors? How did this make you feel? How did you react?
- What should patients or families who feel unheard by doctors do?
- What can doctors do to ensure that their patients feel heard without overextending themselves?
- What can medical systems do to ensure patients feel heard?

THE PERFECT DOCTOR

A Comfortable Silence

•

Amisha Patel

"Is it my fault? What happens next?" A patient asked after being told he had stage IV lung cancer. He sat gently reclined in the hospital's sofa bed with his concerned wife next to him. They held hands tightly as they told me, again, and again, that he had never smoked. That was all they could say. It was all they knew about lung cancer and their only tangible defense.

While I was prepared to take his vitals and gather a complete history, I had not expected to find myself in such a sensitive moment. His diagnosis had been disclosed to him preemptively without much detail. I froze. This was my very first time seeing a patient on my own, and I instantly felt insecure about my ability to help. The idea of death had always felt so abstract and remote to me, but for them, it was known and imminent. It was a conversation waiting to happen.

Almost instinctively, I mentioned that I was just the student and that the attending would be able to answer their questions more completely. It was an easy escape, but quite honestly, it felt incredibly rushed and disingenuous. My history taking was as weak as my initial response to the patient and his wife. I fumbled my way through the questions that did not even seem important at this point, and the physical exam I did felt equally inconsequential. The only thing left to do now was thank them and step out but that, too, did not feel right.

Instead, I placed my stethoscope on the table and sat down on the metal stool next to the bed. I took the man's other hand in mine, took a deep breath, and apologized for not being able to offer more clarity. We sat there quietly for a few moments. There was a sense of trust that filled the room and overpowered any need for small talk. The silence paused the overwhelming reality and let everyone process the moment.

Slowing down was the exact opposite of what I initially knew to do, but it created space and support for the patient and his wife. I understood then that I did not need to have all the answers to be a part of their well-being. I stayed for a few moments longer, and we waited for the oncologist together, holding hands, solaced by the silence. •

Thought questions:
- Are you comfortable with silence? Why or why not?
- Can you think of a moment in which silence has helped you?
- How much is too much silence? How do you know?
- How do you decide when to use or not use silence as a tool in a conversation or medical encounter?

THE PERFECT DOCTOR

Eyes That See

•

Anna Delamerced

It's been months, but I still think of you.
The way you laid in your mother's arms,
Breathing intermittently
Skin like translucent paper
Eyes fully closed

The monitor slowed down.
I counted breaths
One, two, three, four, five

The chaplain knocked on the door, entered this room
Already crowded with strangers in blue masks
Your mother sat in the rocking chair, cradling you, still.
Supplies for the baptism were set on the table:
A glass dish, a vial of water, a soft cloth.
The room quieted down as the rites were said.

Your father looked on, holding your mother's hands.
Tears began to pool in her eyes
Then started to stream down her cheeks
A forest creek under a cloud of rain

The sound of the monitor beeped
One, two, three, four
Signaling when life was ending

Your mother, her eyes, how the tears chased down
The pain of dreams deferred

My heart twisted into a knot, beating harder and harder
Throat dry, hands clammy.
A river of emotion pushing against the dam.
I wanted to cry, but was I allowed to?

One by one we left the room, leaving your parents
To hold you in their arms, still.
The door was closed, work resumed.
Pagers went off. Phone calls made.
Document the time of death.
The morning hours blurred as rounds continued.

Later that day I walked in the garden
Wondering what the color of his eyes were—
Dark brown, chocolate, or hazel like his mother's?
This time, I let the river break the dam
Leveling the waters once more •

Thought questions:
- Is it okay for doctors to cry with patients? When is it appropriate and when is it not?
- People who work in medicine often have to finish their work before they can process their own emotions. Is this healthy and/or sustainable? Is there an alternative? If so, what is it?
- Would it have helped or hurt this patient's family if the writer cried in their presence?

Burnout

•

stopping the fall before it ends

The Puck

•

Joanne Wilkinson

If I were the perfect doctor, I would love talking to people. I wouldn't mind if people needed extra time, or cried a lot during the visit, or told their story in a series of concentric narrative circles that required a lot of backtracking and hitting the delete button while I typed. I would be a little sad when the last patient walked out the door, wishing I could spend more time with people who always seemed to be sad, or sick, or upset, and seemed to want it to be my problem to solve.

Instead, I finish each clinic feeling like I've been bludgeoned with a baseball bat, because even though I genuinely like my patients and find that my interactions with them have widened and enriched my life experience, I honestly can't get myself peppy for one more person at the end of the day sometimes. I have fantasies about working in one of those jobs where you just type in your cubicle and don't talk to anyone.

If I were the perfect doctor, I would not mind at all that the electronic medical record only works half the time. Or that it has all these pop-ups that demand the primary care physician click seven or ten or thirteen buttons. Or that I'm also supposed to update the problem list, add the high complexity codes, successfully level and bill the visit, document everything in the note, order the prescriptions and referrals correctly and close the encounter within a few hours of the visit. While seeing a patient every fifteen minutes. I would never get frustrated or want to tell someone that the charting and typing alone takes more than fifteen minutes. Each time. I would not mind waiting for a long time on hold at CVS, or an even longer time on hold with the insurance company, trying to get something covered that a patient needs, and I would definitely not mind when the pharmacist or the operator or the "peer" in the peer review process called me "Joanne" and assumed I was a secretary or a nurse. This is honestly not surprising that they would think that since most of my time—more than half—is actually spent doing secretarial work. A perfect doctor would not mind this.

But I do. I feel deeply resentful about all of this—not because secretarial work is bad, but because it pains me to work in a career field so deeply illogical that it is paying me doctor wages to click boxes and wait on hold. The system that set up this ridiculousness doesn't seem like it could possibly be saving me money on my health insurance, for example, or helping maximize the match on my retirement contributions. I'm just saying.

I once read an interview with a hockey goalie who said that when things were stressful and everyone was taking shots on goal, that he felt like everything slowed down and got quiet and the puck got really big and that was all he focused on. Every once in a while, when I'm in a room with a patient, my imperfect self trying to deal with the computer and the coding and all the things, this happens to me. Everything slows down, the patient gets big, the computer gets small, and I can feel everything receding around me as I stop and listen more carefully to the patient. Usually, this happens if they say something like:

You know, it's crazy, my sisters all had blood clots in their teens.

Lately, whenever I run for the bus, I get this feeling like there's an elephant on my chest.

It feels like there's a curtain that comes down over my eyes.

If I were the perfect doctor, I would have been secretly glad about COVID, because I would get to work more hours and do more meaningful work and show society that doctors save lives! I wouldn't mind that I was five hours, seven hours, twelve hours in PPE while my child texted me homework questions from the kitchen table, sitting alone with their feet kicking the legs of the high stool, waiting for me to come home. It would all be worth it and I wouldn't think for a moment about my child or my laundry or my groceries because I was Saving Lives.

Somehow, if I were the perfect doctor, I would also prioritize self-care. You can't take good care of others if you neglect your own health! So, while I was pulling off the miracle of the loaves and fishes with the minutes in my clinic and charting all the high complexity codes and getting all the prior authorizations done, I would also find time to meditate every day and go to yoga, because that's what the perfect physicians do. Never mind that I get my stress out by sweating on a Peloton ride and writing novels. It's been made clear to me, from all the emails and Instagram ads I get, that I'm supposed to be relaxing by doing yoga. And after that, I would eat only healthy foods. And get all of my own cancer screening tests done on time. Not cancel my colonoscopy six times because of COVID and having to work extra hours to cover other doctors' shifts. We don't talk about that. I'm pretty sure that you can take good care of your patients while—and in most cases only because—you completely neglect your own health, typing patient notes late into the night and in the early morning hopped up on Diet Coke, sitting down to a meal on a plate with another person only a handful of times per month. No one wants to think of their doctor as someone who is eating a Ding Dong in the back room before they Purell their way in to see you with a bright smile, so let's just agree that perfect doctors don't do that.

If I were the perfect physician, I would be unimaginably tired, and probably sick, so when I finally dragged myself to my own doctor's office, here is what I would be hoping to see:

Someone who looks at me, and sees me.
Someone who asks me questions about my life and gets to know me.
Someone who listens to what I have to say and incorporates it into the plan.
Someone who makes a plan with me and names a time to see me again.
Someone who gives the impression, at least, that they know who I am, and remember me, and care about my health.

And if I say something that makes them want to stop and listen, then the computer will get small, and time will stop, and they will listen.

If they can do that, then I don't care if they ate a Ding Dong on their way in here. I don't care if they don't finish their notes in the session or if they hate yoga. In my book, they are the perfect doctor. •

Thought questions:
- Is it possible to be the kind of doctor who checks all the boxes and is attentive to patients? If so, how?
- The author of this piece highlights the discordance between the business of medicine and its values. What are some ways you have seen the two diverge? What are some ways to reconnect the practice of medicine with its values?
- Have you ever felt at odds with inefficiency that gets in the way of you doing your work? What can be done to address it?

Self-Care and Surgical Training: The Transformative Journey of Becoming a Mother

•

Rebecca Lynn Williams-Karnesky

"Do you have time to see a behavioral health counselor for a few minutes?" the midwife asked as I wiped my eyes with a tissue and tried to surreptitiously blow my nose under my mask.

I looked at my watch. "I have a case at noon, so I guess I have a couple minutes." I replied.

The provider sat there silently for a few seconds staring at me before replying. "So, you're just going to go operate on someone right now?" she asked with a hint of surprise and disbelief.

"Yes?" I answered, not quite knowing what else to say.

At the time, I didn't even think about checking to see if someone else could cover the case. I was sure I already knew the answer—that no one else would be available. Besides, I reasoned, that's just not what surgery residents do.

•

Reflecting on this scene, which occurred at a postpartum visit less than two months after my first child was born while I was a fourth-year surgical trainee, I see an overwhelmed new mother, scared of letting down those around her. I see someone who was so concerned about maintaining her footing as a competent surgery resident that she couldn't ask for a break or for help. Watching this scene in my mind, it is easy for me to understand now why all the emotions I had been burying deep inside so I could continue to function from day to day bubbled up to the surface and erupted in a flood of tears and snot at the small provocation of my medical provider asking how I was doing.

•

BURNOUT

Before I became a mother, if you asked me to describe the perfect surgeon, I would describe someone who was meticulous, efficient, clinically knowledgeable, technically adept, dexterous, and—perhaps above all—self-sacrificing and endlessly devoted to the care of their patients. As a medical student, the breadth and depth of general surgery resonated deeply with me. I loved the singular focus and technicality of the operating room, as well as the unique and intimate relationships that surgeons had with their patients. I saw the long hours that the community surgeons I trained with worked, and as a student I emulated them, coming in to work before the sun rose and leaving after dark—or the next day if I was on call. I was full of vigor and grit, and I loved the challenge.

In my early years as a surgical trainee, I continued my dogged devotion to putting work above all else. I felt it was my responsibility to know every detail about every patient on the service list, even if they were being followed by someone else. I often tried to be the first person on my service in the hospital and the last to leave. I prided myself on my tireless enthusiasm for service to the care of my patients and the team. I was afraid of failing, and I tried to project competency by working hard, by pushing myself to my limit.

•

I got pregnant just before starting my fourth clinical year of surgical training, just after the COVID-19 pandemic hit. I had just completed two non-clinical research years and was about to re-enter my surgical training as a chief on most of the services I would be rotating on. I was struggling with the transition back into full-time clinical work while simultaneously trying to prepare for the life transition that would be occurring in a few short months when my child was born. I felt overwhelmed by self-doubt, fear of making a mistake, and the hormones surging through my body.

Because of this, I worked twice as hard to maintain a façade of competency. I never asked to scrub out of a case. When I was assigned eight-hour cases at 38 weeks pregnant, I just wore compression stockings and hoped that my baby's kidneys would be okay with my abysmal fluid intake for the day. I worked a 24-hour call four days before my child was born. I never asked for an exemption or to be removed from the call-pool. In fact, I was one of the administrative chief residents and I helped make the call schedule that forced me to work that shift. At the time, I felt like putting myself on a 24-hour call in my gravid state would be recognized as an obvious act of devotion to my chosen profession. Everyone could finally see how far I was willing to go to be the perfect surgical trainee.

Perhaps the most ridiculous part about my behavior during that late stage of my pregnancy is that I've always been a vocal champion for well-being in medicine. I started practicing Zen Buddhism seriously in medical school and found many benefits from my mindfulness practice. I saw mindfulness as a tool that could help other medical trainees, so I created a course on mindfulness for medical students. Ultimately, the course became a mandatory part of the surgery clerkship. I also worked with a senior resident to help create and run a wellness curriculum for our surgical residency program, lobbying for protected educational time for trainees to learn about ergonomics, personal finance, self-compassion, and meditation. I wrote papers and gave talks on the importance of provider wellbeing, job satisfaction, retention in medicine, and patient outcomes.

Beyond my curricular efforts, I made sure to reassure others—especially medical students and residents that were junior to me—that it was okay to take care of themselves. Yes! They could leave early. (I could double check that all the morning labs were ordered.) Yes! They could have an extra day off tomorrow because they stayed late yesterday. (I could cover the floor and the operating room. It's easy because I'm a senior, right?) Yes! They should hand off the pager to someone else to spend time with their family who is in town this weekend. (Oh, the other intern is sick? Then yes! They could just hand the pager to me!)

•

Early in surgical training, I think I did a reasonable job of using mindfulness as a tool to help me attend to my wellbeing. But as I progressed in training, I became more and more caught up in the myth of the self-sacrificing surgeon that I truly felt powerless to address my own needs. I felt like taking time to attend to myself—taking time away from my duties as a surgical trainee—was selfish. There was always something more important to attend to, some deadline to meet, some project to complete, some shift to cover. Even when I found out I was pregnant, I felt afraid to tell people about it, worried they might not think I was 'tough enough' to carry out my daily responsibilities.

After my child was born, my understanding of personal wellbeing began to change. Becoming a mother helped me see that I needed to take care of myself to be able to take care of my child and my family. Recognizing the benefits of breastfeeding, I asked to scrub out of cases to pump so I could keep my milk supply up. Before my child was born, I bought wearable breast-pumps, planning to use my pumping time to multitask while catching up on charting. Once I was back to work from maternity leave, when I did take breaks to pump, I found that my milk let-down happened much more readily if I just looked at pictures of my new baby, so that's what I did instead of staring at the electronic medical record. If I could, I would even try to have a short video-chat with my husband and baby, because that was what really nourished me. When I took 24-hour call, my husband would drive to the hospital in the evening so I could nurse. The hard separation I had created in my mind between work and life began to soften.

What I also noticed, was that as I allowed myself some grace, and attended to my own needs—physical and emotional—I was able to take better care of those around me. Spending time away from work and with my family, expanded the compassion I had for my patients and their families. I was in awe of every new accomplishment of my child: a smile, a coo, shaking a rattle. My child was a magnificent, unique being, with inherent value. I started seeing my patients in this way as well. I thought about them being someone's child, and I experienced their suffering through the eyes of a mother. It even allowed me to start to hold a sliver of that compassion for myself. The profound transition of becoming a mother gave new meaning to my role as a healer.

•

Unfortunately, the emotional postpartum visit with my midwife wasn't the catalyst for me to miraculously transform into someone who has self-care, motherhood, and surgical training all figured out. I continued to struggle with postpartum depression and the need to appear competent and hard-working. The idea of self-sacrifice and neglect of my own needs were still tied up in my conception of what it meant to be a perfect surgeon. But it was one step on the journey of awakenings to the need for self-acceptance and balance. •

Thought questions:
- Can you think of a time when you did not "practice what you preach," like the author who created wellness curricula but did not attend to her own wellness? What was your reason for doing so? Would you do something differently if you were to do it again? How and why?
- Should a surgeon prioritize their patients over their family? What are the consequences if they do, and if they do not?
- What support systems need to be in place at work and/or at home to cope with the sometimes conflicting needs of patients and a doctor's own family?

THE PERFECT DOCTOR

Tethered

•

Harika Kottakota

I feel the tugs begin
in a languid crescendo
before the familiar
eruption of dread
prickles across my skin,
diving into every bony crypt

a slipped stitch
  a stubborn IV
    a murmur unheard

surely, You will see
past my collapsing veneer,
how my gait is now a trudge
across the linoleum floor,
the slight tremble in my hands
as I reach for your pulse

if only You could hear
the erratic fugue
between my temples
as I clench the fraying
white threads
of this leaden coat

how I've endured this
coy and insidious affair
of crisp, waxing-waning
waves of worry
crashing against me

BURNOUT

Your eyes nonetheless
glimmer
with a grave hope
that I carry
all the answers,
all the remedies
we both seek •

Thought questions:
- Think of a time when you made a mistake. How did it feel in your body?
- Should doctors share how they feel with patients? Why or why not?
- What helps you overcome self-doubt?

THE PERFECT DOCTOR

Silence

•

Sapana Adhikari

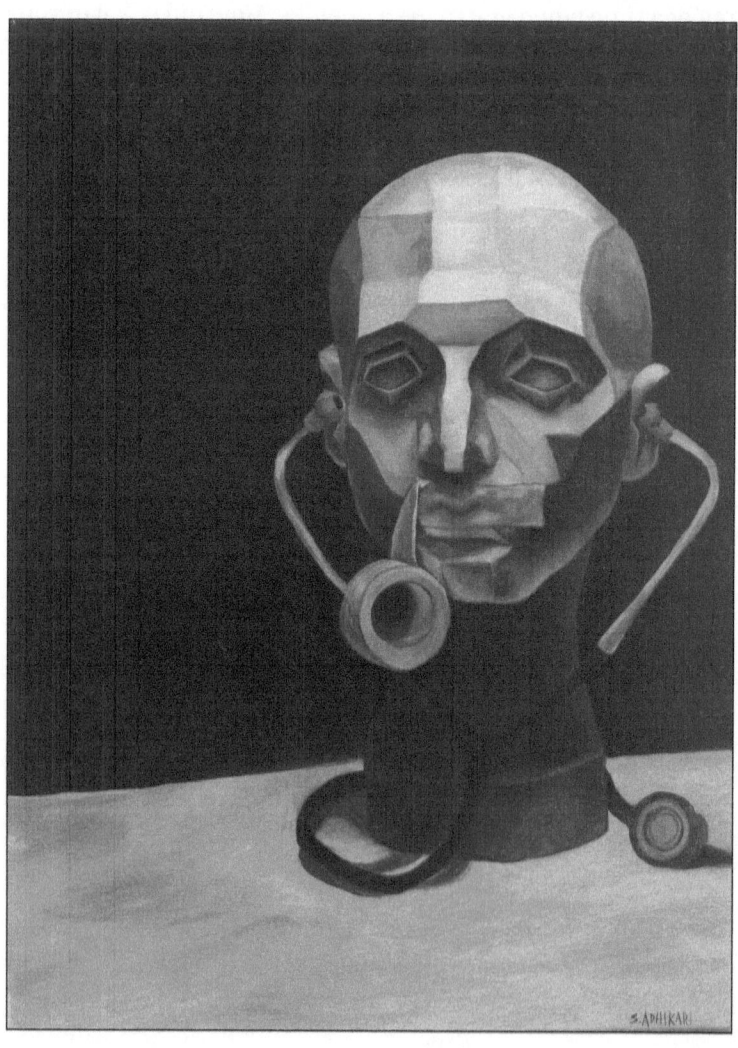

The physician in today's society has much to say but often feels unable or afraid to speak up. The painting depicts a "model" head with perfect proportions, representing the idealized image of a physician. Although the model appears perfect, the viewer subtly notices the medical tape, used to silence the physician. The stethoscope around the neck, in the familiar, yet suffocating way, is strategically perched to the viewer to depict that the physician is listening to what is going on all around, but cannot say a word. •

Thought questions:
- Do you ever feel silenced? If so, by what or who, and how?
- What are some avenues to use your voice? How effective are these avenues at enacting change?
- If you had the ear of a leaders who could affect change in health care, what would you say?
- Is speaking up enough? If not, what kind of action is needed to affect the change you feel is necessary and who's responsibility is the action?

THE PERFECT DOCTOR

No Absences

•

Charlotte Grinberg

During my third year of medical school, I overheard my classmates discussing the policy of two excused absences per six-week clinical rotation. Most students described feeling intensely guilty about taking even one of these excused days off, even if they felt genuinely sick. Others bragged about how few days total they had taken off the whole year. They, myself included, had missed weddings, birthdays, reunions, and funerals. We were celebrating these nonappearances. Loved ones in my life soon started assuming I wouldn't make it to their festivities and milestones. To my husband (who isn't in medicine), the irony was that not only were we nonessential workers, but we were students (paying to learn!). Yet that desire to be fully committed, fully present, and fully self-sacrificing gripped us from the beginning.

My type-A personality helped craft this mindset. It's the same pressure that drove me to always want the perfect test score, write the perfect essay, and create the perfect social interaction. I was saying no to doing things for personal reasons long before medical school. Whereas before medical school I was the exception, during medical school I was surrounded by those who shared an intense commitment to professional development. It further normalized the behavior of putting school and career above everything else.

Some of this desire for perfection in medicine also came from external pressures. Fast forward to intern year, rotating on an inpatient medicine service, with 12-hour long days and no time for structured breaks. I spent half the time on my cell phone during a noon learning conference trying to coordinate purchasing flights with my husband to visit our families in France. The chief resident came up to me after the lecture, and said "Hey, try to look more engaged in the future." Never had I received words of affirmation or support from this person. I repeated those words of disappointment in my head for the rest of the week. It was normal that residents who stayed hours past their shifts, or never called in sick, were described and perceived as more dedicated to the work.

Throughout all my clinical training and practice, I've experienced this deeply entrenched and pervasive mindset that the perfect doctor is the doctor who is always present and available: the doctor that is fully committed to the hospital, to the team, to the work, to the schedule, to the patient. Of course, hard work is necessary to being a good provider—but hard work doesn't have to mean 24/7 availability.

As I've challenged myself to overcome my nature and to value the personal and the familial, to experience the humanness and vulnerability of life, I've felt the pressure to hide my life outside the hospital. When I had a second trimester miscarriage as a third-year medical student and asked to take a few days off to recover, I was told by the clerkship administrator I would receive a failing grade for my rotation. I took the Step 3 exam within a week of that miscarriage to remain on the expected school timeline, sitting through many multiple-choice questions about pregnancy.

When I had two kids during residency and exclusively breastfed them, I navigated pumping in secrecy. I would rush to pump in an on-call room after excusing myself from rounds to use the bathroom, and if I was feeling particularly brave, I would sneak to the hospital lobby where my husband would be waiting with my son to nurse. When I had family members navigate end of life care and death, I didn't share these deaths with my coworkers and prioritized getting back to work as soon as possible. I am eternally grateful for my husband who, despite my resistance, purchased tickets for me to fly to France to attend the funeral of my aunt when she died from lung cancer. At the time, I thought the test I had to study for was more important. I don't remember the test. I do remember keeping vigil for my aunt and my cousins who lost their mom.

I now recognize that these "hidden" experiences have actually made me a better doctor. With each personal milestone and hardship, I've developed more empathy and more presence for my clinical care. I connect better with patients, I understand their experiences more, and I allow myself to acknowledge the complexities of life.

My favorite attending during residency was a cardiologist with four little kids. He was the first doctor in my medical training who openly displayed, and even embraced, the realities of balancing clinical and personal life. Not infrequently would he be on the phone with his wife figuring out last-minute school and extracurricular logistics, or at the bank ATM withdrawing money for babysitters. He didn't seem to worry that we saw the messiness, and it deepened my respect for him. I also learned from him how to thoughtfully manage patients with heart failure and ischemic heart disease. He made me believe that I too could have a big family and be a dedicated clinician. He normalized that some days are really hard logistically. When he accidentally stumbled upon me in a conference room on the verge of tears after a nanny fiasco, he took a seat at the table. Rather than deny my situation, I let him know I was struggling. He shared his many childcare disaster stories and made phone calls to help me find a childcare solution.

Imagine if we practiced in a health care system where the perfect doctor was one that comfortably and openly acknowledged the nuances of life, both inside and outside the hospital. I try to be this doctor now... with my kids either laughing or yelling in the background when I take hospice evening and weekend calls from home. I have looked for supportive colleagues who genuinely don't pass judgment when I need to leave early to get to a kid's dentist or doctor's appointment, and they feel comfortable asking me for the same assistance. We know that we all more than make up for it with extra hours after bedtime. I still have to work hard to dispel the narrative in my mind that this makes me less worthy of being a doctor and a coworker. But it's worth it to feel less resentment towards my job, more closeness with my patients and coworkers, and to be there for more of life's moments. •

Thought questions:
- Are there any downsides to supervising physicians being honest with trainees about their life outside of medicine?
- Who benefits and who is harmed when a doctor is always available to patients?
- Fact: 24/7 availability of clinicians is necessary. Can clinicians be available for patients 24/7 and still have a life? If so, what measures need to be in place for this to be sustainable?

BURNOUT

Do No Self-Harm

•

Palak Shah

I became an expert at reading my colleagues' foreheads. The pandemic shielded our mouths and our noses, wrapped our heads, adorned our bodies from neck to toe with protective gowns. My eyes naturally gravitated to the only part I was able to recognize in the colleagues around me. I found myself trying to decipher foreheads when words often failed us. The ICU attending was one such colleague that I'd had many encounters with, enough to anticipate her needs and glean information from her tone. Three raised lines across her forehead signified worry, a furrowing in the center of her forehead meant anger or exasperation. One night in particular, the top of her head was smooth, with beads of perspiration collecting on the edges like dew collects in the dawn under the weight of all her gear. There was nary a crinkle; she was unbothered, almost calm. However, her calmness was not reminiscent of a placid lake but more like that preceding a storm.

The intensivist was often a lighthouse in rough waters, directing her colleagues through difficult clinical situations and augmenting morale. Now, however, her eyes lacked luster, her mind seemingly swirling in an echo chamber of defeat. The look on her face, or rather the absence of emotion, was one that I knew all too well: a push-and-pull collateral between numbness and vulnerability, feeling nothing and everything simultaneously. Similar to the intensivist who I saw become a fragment of her former self, I, too, unraveled under the weight of all that was asked of us. We were caregivers first, but our roles also evolved into being social support systems for patients whose family members were unable to be present bedside. Our clinical acumen became stifled by all that we did not know, resolutely holding onto interventions with the faintest plausibility of success. How do you cope when your knowledge is failing and your faith wavering? When you're forced to make a home out of a barricade?

During the end of every shift, on my way home, I would pass a billboard for a nursing program that very proudly proclaimed, "It's amazing to be needed." Initially, I would feel gratified reading it. I would be remiss if I failed to mention that this sense of pride was accompanied with a certain tinge of conceit due to the virtuosity bestowed upon the health care field at times. As the pandemic surged, that pride, ultimately, dissipated into anger, which then metamorphosed into a general feeling of inadequacy. The pandemic reinforced at the end of my residency what should have been cured throughout the three years: the ever-daunting imposter syndrome.

We start medical school with a thunderous proclamation of "do no harm." However, there is no mention of how we minimize self-harm; no broaching upon how we nurture self-awareness; no allusion to how we prevent burnout by prioritizing self-care. These were omissions that made the Hippocratic oath seem incomplete: Our mental and physical health as caregivers was not just an afterthought, but rather inconsequential and sometimes an inconvenience.

At the time I was experiencing this emotional disassociation, I did not have a name for it. It was not until I started business school and took an ethics class in leadership that I found a diagnosis; it was in the hinterland of *moral fatigue* where I was forced to contend with my own mental health that acted as a barrier from delivering good care. However, rather than feeling relieved at having gained some insight into my own plight, I felt a need to hide what I was going through. Acquiescing to a defeatist attitude was deemed more noble than doing something about it.

I carried on privately trying to ameliorate my sense of well-being in relation to my role as healer. Much like non-adherence is as dangerous as over-utilization of medication, I found that empathy must also be dispensed in equitable levels and refilled regularly to avoid burnout, particularly when we succumb to the limitations of science and of self. Additionally, I became adept at creating a chorus of like-minded trusted colleagues that helped me recognize symptoms of burnout when we find ourselves straying from our mental and emotional homeostasis. More importantly, I employed mindfulness in daily practice to help me understand the value of introspection and the courage to accept that one provider cannot bear it all, despite systemic expectations.

Resiliency is a feat we often preach but never teach. This serves to be detrimental in a field where more answers inspire more questions and the chasm between what we know and do not know only widens. However, perfection in medicine is not dashed because we fall, it is upheld because we rise knowing we will fall again. Learning how to cope between the fall and the rise can make all the difference in saving not only patients' lives, but the caregiver's as well. •

Thought questions:
- How can resiliency be taught?
- How do you refill your empathy?
- What is the "organizational prescription" for moral fatigue?

Doctors as Patients

•

(im)perfect encounters
from the other side

How You Failed Me

•

Maya Sorini

Dear Dr. A,

We met when I was 22, though I am sure you do not remember me. I was already on opioids when you came into the emergency room where I lay, and I must have seemed docile and clueless. My hair was a nest of sweaty tangles from my helmet, I was still wearing riding breeches, and my hospital gown lay over my chest like a blanket. There was a beautiful girl sitting with me, my roommate, who asked about your UCLA lanyard, since she is from LA. You ignored her.

The emergency room resident and attending had just finished their exam. The resident had tenderly pressed an ultrasound probe to my shoulder blade to see inside the joint space. The resident narrated what he saw to the attending, a doctor I had worked with several times and greatly respected, who agreed that there was blood and fat inside my shoulder. This would imply that a broken bone was spilling marrow into the space, which would account for the sensation that my arm was slowly being torn off. Before the Percocet kicked in, I was in so much pain I could not finish my sentences. With the pills in my system, I was deep underwater.

They had already taken X-rays, but I know you did not look at them before you came to examine me. I know that because the break was visible on the X-rays, which the outpatient orthopedics fellow showed me two days later when asking why I had been put through a CT scan.

It was a Friday night in St. Louis, a beautiful February day that felt more like April, and I know you were swamped with traumas. In the waiting room post-Percocet, I had tenderly assured the parents of a gunshot wound victim that their son was getting great care from the trauma team (my coworkers and bosses). You were probably getting paged every hour, at least, to some victim of violent crime or severe accident. I was one of the minor cases you saw in between those splintered femurs and open-book pelvic fractures. I know that because I spent thousands of hours in your emergency room researching trauma patients. Months later, I would stand in an OR with you, pretending that I did not know your face as you pinned a femur.

You came into my room at around 1 a.m. I had fallen off the horse at about 2 p.m. but had not arrived at the ER until 6 p.m. (That is another story, and not your fault.) I had waited in anguish for three hours before my roommate arrived with dinner and discovered me rocking back and forth and weeping in silence. It was all I could do to speak a few words through the pain. She walked to the nurse's station at the front of the waiting room and demanded I be given pain medicine. Once those opioids hit my system, the night became a wash of color and sound. I was finally let into a room at about midnight. My shoulder was very painful, but I was deep under the medicine and growing exhausted.

You said very little when you came in the room, but asked me to sit up and move aside my gown so you could look at my left shoulder. You moved your hands over my back for about twenty seconds, before pulling my gown back up and stepping away. You told me that you doubted I had dislocated my shoulder or that anything was broken. You said that you probably would not come back once you left, though you would review my CT scan, and that a nurse could help me get a sling and schedule an outpatient appointment for me sometime that week. Then you breezed out of the room, onto more interesting cases.

What you failed to see was that I was more interesting than you thought. I had a rare posterior dislocation (you know, the kind that account for less than 5% of all dislocations and usually occur in the elderly or professional athletes?) that probably only happened because of an underlying hypermobility condition. You missed a diagnosis you will probably never see again during your residency training because you ignored me.

I understand your quickness. I know your life is busy, have seen one of your co-residents break down at the workload of ortho traumas that they must cover in the ED, but your brusqueness was an embarrassment. When the CT came back and showed my broken humerus and the growing space in my joint as fluid pushed on the bones, the ED resident returned and told me in a gentle voice what had happened. He had been right, there was a break, and I had been right, there had been a dislocation which I had somehow re-located myself after getting back on the horse that had thrown me.

He spoke softly, since it was nearly 4 a.m. and I was drifting in and out of a drugged sleep. He told me about the prescription for more Percocet he was writing and even took the time to detail how many days I could take the pills before physical dependence set in. You never returned, though you should have been the expert in charge of my care.

You failed me because you did not care. You could have paid attention to my roommate's pleasantries, even if you found them tiresome. You could have said, "I do not think your shoulder is broken, which is good because that means it will heal more quicky, and I'm sorry I won't be able to stop back in later. Just to be sure, I want to get a CT scan to get a better picture of the bones. I hope you feel better soon." I used a stopwatch; that took me 19 seconds to read aloud. I know you were probably hungry, your feet probably hurt, someone may have died under your hands that afternoon, believe me, I know. I know how it feels to be so tired you think you could melt into the floors and disappear.

You acted like you thought my condition, my pain, were beneath you. You chose not to take the time to really see me or treat me. You were a young physician, you failed me that night, and I forgive you. If you will allow this piece of advice: the next time you want to roll your eyes at a patient in pain and pass her off to a nurse, I implore you, spend thirty seconds longer in that room. That way, she will not remember you as I do: as an aloof asshole who misdiagnosed me.

All my best,
Posterior dislocation of left humerus, initial encounter •

Thought questions:
- What could have been running through the surgeon's mind during his interaction with the writer?
- Have you ever been a patient and felt disrespected? Describe the incident and what you did about it.
- If you haven't already, consider writing a letter to a person who disrespected you. You can write it for yourself and then throw it away. Or, you may choose to find a way to respectfully communicate your feelings with that person. If you do choose to communicate your feelings, it's often helpful to consider your intentions for doing so, use "I" statements, and sleep on it before you send.
- If you are/were a doctor, how would you feel getting such a letter? Have you ever received feedback about your actions towards another person that was unexpected? How did you cope with this feedback?

The Other Place

•

Danielle Wilfand

I'm not sure why, but what I remember most about the waiting room was a floor-to-ceiling fish tank that ran through the center, bisecting it in two. There were all sorts of fish in it: orange ones, yellow ones, blue ones. I made eye contact with a black and white striped fish which just as quickly flitted away, leaving only my reflection staring back at me. I was surprised by how small I looked, pale. Alone. No, I was not truly alone, my mom was seated near me. I had convinced her to let me buy a caramel Frappuccino from Starbucks on the way in and I still had it clutched in my hand. I didn't know it then, but this would become a sort of ritual each time I would need to come back here. My eyes wandered around the room and settled on two children seated at a small table scribbling in a coloring book. They were laughing amongst themselves, energetic and carefree, but it stood out oddly in a place like this, seeming almost unnatural.

I came to the sudden realization that I was probably the oldest patient there. I had just turned 14 a few months before and was starting high school soon. In all that time, I had never been to a children's hospital. I had always been relatively healthy—a few earaches, courses of antibiotics, trips to the pediatrician. Never more than that. But my last visit to the pediatrician was different., The nurse whisked me away for a bunch of tests as soon as I came in. With one eyebrow raised, my pediatrician examined the results, then handed me a referral to a pediatric gastroenterologist at the major children's hospital in the city.

A medical assistant in printed scrubs materialized from behind a set of doors and called my name. I got up and followed her back, my mom close behind me. The blood pressure cuff squeezed my arm and she asked me some questions. My date of birth? Was I in any pain? I gave her one-word replies. A new room, more fish. This time they were in the form of stickers placed all over the walls. There were even some on the ceilings. I would later learn that this part of the hospital was called River (and I would come to know it well over the next few years). I took a seat at the edge of the exam table swinging my legs in the empty space, trying to keep the fear from clawing up into my throat, from choking me entirely. I looked up at the fish. I was drowning.

A knock rang out through the room and the doctor walked in. His navy blue scrubs were well-worn, lived in. In the years to come, I don't think I ever saw him in anything but that pair of scrubs. A couple of multi-colored pens protruded from the breast pocket and he grasped one as he took a seat across from me. He asked me what had brought me here and I told him. The words rolled off my tongue so quickly and easily and I felt embarrassed. It was as if once the dam had burst, the flood of water would not stop. I told him everything. The pain, the blood, the exhaustion. How I could taste iron in my mouth and every time I stood up, black spots would flash in front of my eyes. After I finished speaking, he sat quietly for a few minutes, hands resting in his lap.

"Have you ever heard of a disease called ulcerative colitis?"

I nodded. I had (having done a few unfortunate Google searches prior to my appointment).

"What does this mean for me?"

What will my life look like now? What kind of future will I have?

He paused for a little while. "When I was 12, I was diagnosed with juvenile diabetes," He said, pointing to the insulin pumped clipped onto his pocket. "It hasn't always been easy, but through proper management, I've been able to lead the life I wanted, even become a physician."

I didn't know it at the time, but that moment would completely change the course of my life in more ways than one. It was like all of a sudden, something clicked and an event that could have been devastating instead morphed into the catalyst which set me on the path to becoming a doctor. I wanted to be what my doctor had been for me in that moment for others, and that became the singular driving force that propelled me through the next ten years of my life.

•

The stage was almost impossibly grand. It was in the main auditorium of a music hall, its walls lined with intricately carved golden panels, bouquets of roses surrounding the stage. Roses that would eventually be given to us. A lone podium stood in the center of it all, the crest of the medical school etched in gold at its base. As the dean entered, surrounded by an entourage of long white coats, we rose from our seats, one hand raised, chanting the oath we had written together. Almost 10 years had passed since I was diagnosed with ulcerative colitis and it hadn't been easy, but my journey led me here—to my white coat ceremony, marking the beginning of my first year of medical school.

I stood in line with my fellow classmates, and when the dean of the medical school called my name, I made my way across the stage to the applause of the auditorium. They gave me a white coat, and it didn't change anything. I'm not sure why I thought it would. Maybe something inside of me had thought of it as a symbol that I had conquered the disease, that I had made it to the other side and now it couldn't touch me anymore.

It didn't take long for the cracks to begin to show. The morning of my first anatomy exam I knew something was wrong. I woke up over an hour before my alarm with a dull ache in my head. I went to the bathroom to wash my face and for the first time that morning, I caught sight of myself in the mirror. The whites of my eyes were fully blood red. I couldn't put my finger on why, but something about it sent a chill down my spine. The next day, I realized I couldn't see the screen from my usual seat in lecture, and each following day I had to move up closer and closer until I was in the front row. But I still couldn't see. What I initially thought was a headache spurred on by stress or sleep deprivation slowly morphed into what felt like a fist pressing against the back of my left eye.

The next day, I went to the emergency ophthalmology clinic. The waiting room walls were gray, the chairs were gray. I couldn't see much of anything more. An elderly couple sat across from me—I couldn't see their faces, but it looked like one had grasped the other's hand and was cradling it tenderly. Someone called my name, and I followed them back to another small gray room. I stared into the machine and watched the flickering dots until they disappeared into the darkness at the edges of my vision. The room was so dim I could barely see my hands trembling in my lap. The doctor came in and shined a bright light in my eyes. As he was leaving, he turned around.

"There's something wrong with your brain."

Then left, the door clicking closed behind him. Left in the dark, it was like something inside of me broke and I cried and cried and cried.

•

It moved on from my eyes, attacked my feet and hands. Still, no one knew what was wrong. I tried to stay in school, but my body was failing me. When I walked through the high glass doors of the medical school on my way to class, it was as if I was truly seeing everything for the first time. I looked around and realized how much I didn't belong. Being a physician had been my dream for so long. I had grasped onto it with everything I had and refused to let go. But I realized that in my dream, the me I had constructed in my head was different from the one that really existed. I edited out the hospitalizations, the infections, the illness. The me that I pictured as a doctor was healthy, and at that moment I realized so was the doctor that everyone around me had pictured. I was bluntly confronted by the fact that I was not like my classmates. When they were studying, lining up research opportunities, and shadowing in the hospital, I was hopping from one doctor's appointment to another, desperately trying to survive. My body did not allow me to be like them.

I couldn't be the image of perfection that was expected of me. I limped up the stairs to my small group discussion, unbeknownst to me for the last time that year. We sat around the table and discussed the case before us—a patient with chronic myeloid leukemia. He was scared of what would happen if the cancer came back again, if the drugs didn't work. We talked about the case for a while, mechanisms of DNA translocations and oncogenes. I tried to keep up with the conversation, but my mind kept wandering. A stray thought drifted through my mind. I looked more like the patient than I did like my classmates sitting next to me. After that, it became too much, and I couldn't go on anymore. So, I disappeared as if the ground itself had swallowed me up. Deep down I went into the dark and cold. Back to that other place.

There is a place that I know. Not a physical one but equally real, nonetheless. The place in my mind that I would go when I was hospitalized on the River floor of the children's hospital, when I was alone and no one understood what I was going through, and I couldn't do the things I wanted to do. When I was younger, I never had the words to describe it, but I always knew it was there, like an invisible hand on my shoulder. It was very dark and lonely, and sometimes when I went there, it felt like I would never be able to get out again. It was other and othering. When I was an undergrad, I happened upon a book that opened with a quote from Susan Sontag's *Illness as a Metaphor*.

> *Illness is the night side of life, a more onerous citizenship. Everyone who is born holds dual citizenship, in the kingdom of the well and in the kingdom of the sick.*

That was the first time I had ever seen this place put into words. The kingdom of the sick. When I would miss school, all my friends, my teachers, everyone, would ask me: Where do you go when you're not here? Now after all this time, I could tell them. This is where I go.

How does one climb out of the dark? Months had passed since I took a leave of absence from school, and I was healing physically. But still, I was left with so many questions. *Did I even want to return to medicine? Would there ever be a place for me?* I thought back to that appointment all those years ago and why it impacted me the way it did. I realized it was because, in that moment, I felt like someone understood what I was going through, that someone saw the same dark place I had and wanted to show me that there was a way forward.

As I met more people like me, in support groups, in the hospitals I worked in, I realized that in the kingdom of the sick, I was never as alone as I thought. There were others who knew that same place, some who knew it better than I did. And some you'd never think knew it based on how they looked. Medicine and the path to get there often excludes people with disabilities because we often do not—and cannot—fit the narrow mold of what a physician is supposed to look like. The experiences people with disabilities bring to medicine are important because these are the same experiences of our patients. I restarted medical school again the next year. And this time it was different than before. Knowing where they have walked, I could give my patients so much more: that there was a way out of the dark, and even if there wasn't, they were not alone. •

Thought questions:
- Have you been to 'the other place?' If so, describe your experience.
- What helped you move through 'the other place' back to 'the kingdom of life?'
- How can you help others move through?
- Should one's experience with the other place be shared openly or kept private? What are the pros and cons of sharing and keeping it to oneself?

DOCTORS AS PATIENTS

The Mortal Physician

•

Rachel Scheub

"I don't know how you do this." My patient's words rang through my mind throughout the morning. She had just delivered her second child, an impressive and wonderful milestone for anyone, but an even greater challenge for the patient with type 1 diabetes. I disclosed to her that I too share her diagnosis, and her awe that followed at my career choice encompassed my inner feelings about the constant balance between the two roles I play within this hospital. In that moment, I redirected her awe towards her own feat of childbirth, but her words rang through my head.

Throughout my short career in medicine, I have often struggled with how my role as patient fits into my role as a medical student. In a world where I am constantly evaluated, my fear of being a burden to my team has led to a pursuit of perfectionism in controlling a disease that can be unpredictable and difficult to manage. My 5.5 hemoglobin A1c, a normal measure of average blood sugar, and the desire to blend in creates the illusion that I am *different* than other patients with diabetes, but in seven words, my patient reminded me of the struggle we share. On the surface, I am theoretically surrounded by professionals most in tune with disease and the patient experience. On the inside, however, entering the medical world as both a patient and a provider is a cultural shock woven by a fear of demonstrating weakness and an aversion to seeking help.

The insulin pump's triple beep is unrelenting, a purposeful design intended to alert of an impending hypoglycemic doom. With this noble intention, it has subsequently spoken its purpose at the least convenient of times. Mid-exam, I fear it will be perceived as cheating; mid patient encounter, I excuse myself to inhale a bag of fruit snacks in world-record speed; mid-rounds, I sprint to and from the nutrition room before my absence can be detected. The insulin pump blends into the sounds of beeping monitors and beeping pagers, the song of the role of provider continuously competing in a tug of war with the role of patient.

Physicians have struggled for years with the role of self-disclosure in medicine. We have moved toward a culture shift away from the all-knowing physician toward a world where we are allowed to be real humans with real lives. I have watched countless patients relax with the knowledge that their pediatrician has children of their own and can relate to their fears as a parent. Acknowledging that we are all human allows a depth of empathy that would be impossible in a paternalistic world.

When I wonder about how my role as a patient fits into my role as a medical student, I am wondering about the same thing we all have wondered at some point in our careers: How can I be a human and a doctor? The two roles I play in the hospital, patient and provider, became one when I told my patient we struggle with the same disease. Merging the parts of us that define us with our practice of medicine, the titles we carry—patient, partner, parent—fuse with physician and allow us to be human. Instead of balancing and separating my roles, which only fosters anxiety that being a medical student should prevail above all, I can instead be myself—Type 1 diabetes and all—and consequently form stronger connections with my patients that allow me to build trust and provide better care.

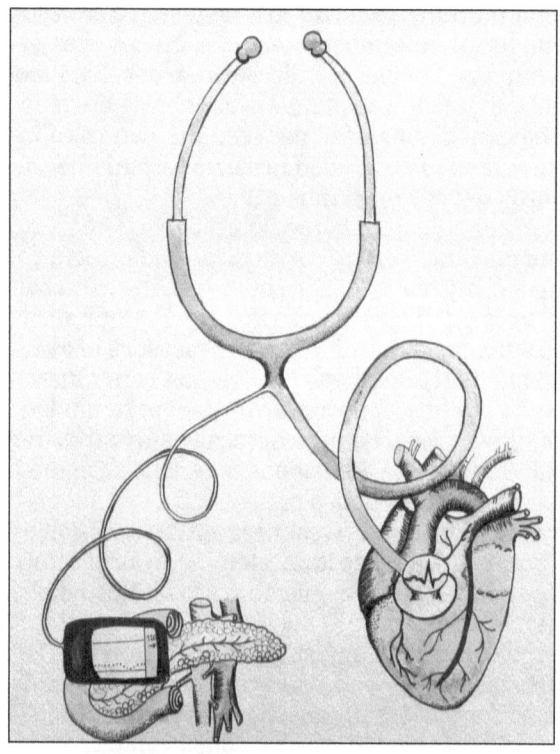

Double Edged Stethoscope: This painting depicts a stethoscope that both leads to a heart and branches off to an insulin pump overlaying a pancreas. It is a visual depiction of my own roles as a medical student and as a patient with type one diabetes. The insulin pump and stethoscope diaphragm are separated in space and connected by the top of the stethoscope, depicting how these roles are both distinct sectors of my life whilst also connected.

DOCTORS AS PATIENTS

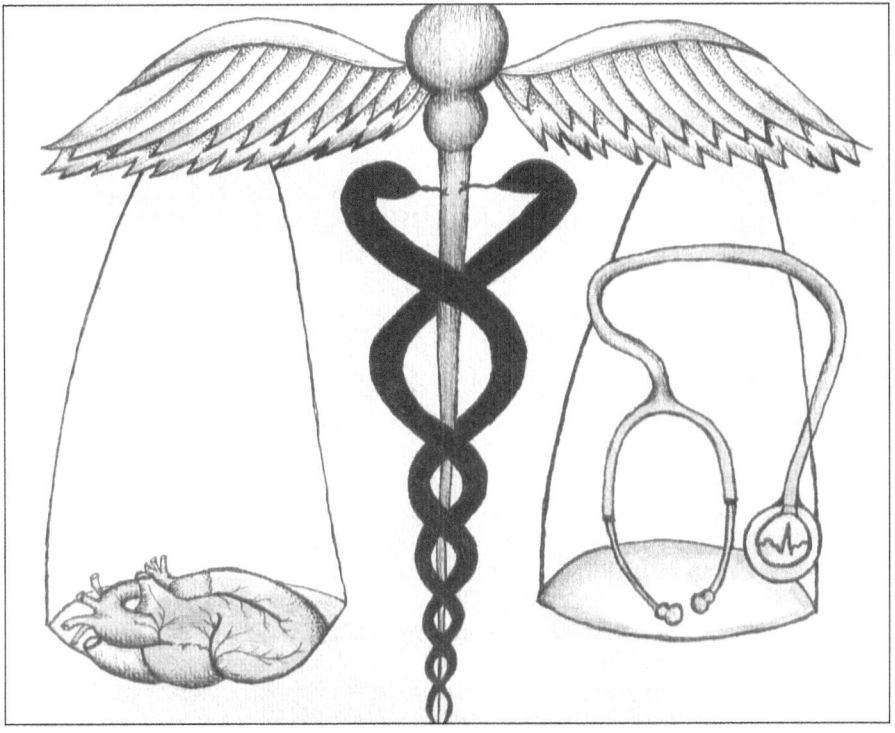

Balance: This painting depicts a scale made from the caduceus, a symbol of medicine, weighing a human heart and a stethoscope. This painting is a direct response to the previous one, in which the idea of "doctor" and "patient" are further separated. It shows the dilemma of balancing taking care of oneself and high performance in this career. •

Thought questions:
- How does the balance between one's own health and work stand out for physicians compared to people in other careers? Are physicians unique, or must other health care professionals and people who work outside of health care cope with this challenge?
- How does the message behind this writing and artwork apply to people without chronic illness?
- Medical licensing and hospital credentialing applications often ask if physicians need "special accommodations" to get their work done. Are these questions necessary? What are the pros and cons of such questions?
- What are some ways in which the medical system can not only provide equitable health care, but also treat its health care workers with equity?

THE PERFECT DOCTOR

Above and Beyond

•

Susie Jiaxing Pan

Growing up, my visits to the doctor's office were among my least favorite activities. Whether it was a simple checkup or a visit to the emergency room, I hated them equally. Maybe it was something about the bleakness of the white walls and white coats that intimidated me. Or the sheer abundance of sharp tools that were apparently for saving, not hurting, that I couldn't rationalize in my head. Or maybe it was the quiet, melancholy murmurs of people lurking in the waiting area who come from all walks of life that pained my heart a little. Or maybe it was the stern authority that radiated from every word and movement of a doctor that sent shivers running down my spine.

How could I possibly feel comfortable expressing my thoughts and pouring out my story to the clinical, blank stare of a white coat? A coat made to conceal the true worries of a medical professional tasked with reassuring the frayed nerves of patients and their families. How could I, an exceptionally imperfect, emotional young adult, possibly become one of these powerful, composed real-life superheroes myself?

In the quest to answer this question, I began thinking about the relationship I have with my own doctor, the person who holds my life in their hands. I found that, ideally, our relationship would be much like a best friend, except with much higher stakes. I hope that my doctor treats me not just as an anatomical subject, not just a checklist of symptoms, not just a medical textbook of examples. Rather, I want my doctor to evaluate my health within the context of my own struggles, for my doctor to realize that my physical wounds stretch beyond their physiological base. I want those external factors in my living situation, like financial instability and family disputes to be considered holistically as factors in my health.

I hope that my doctor's perspective on my health spans more than one dimension. I want there to be a duality in our patient-provider relationship where my doctor sees me for more than my illness and where I see my doctor for more than a job. There is more to each of us as people than the medical circumstance we cross paths in. I want to be recognized with professional courtesy, but without the monotone script. Hearing the same strategic words voiced in a flat tone makes me struggle to feel comfortable in my hospital experience. Above all, I want my doctor to pair my health care concerns with my personal testimonies—to remember that the girl who came in with a scorching fever and a dry cough is the same girl that swims freely at the lake, that travels with her family, that laughs with her friends. The same girl that looks up to her doctor because one day, that's where she sees herself in life.

To view this in a larger scope on a societal level, I believe the majority of patients covet a treatment experience that embraces an accommodating and personal approach. However, this does not appeal to everyone. In terms of feasibility, I am hesitant that a doctor can be everything every patient wants. The hedonic treadmill is inevitable and unless a doctor tailors his/her care specifically to each patient, which is a titanic task, the idea seems neither likely nor realistic.

Regardless, it remains critical for a doctor to be agile and adaptive to patient preferences, especially having the awareness to exhibit emotional intelligence during those interactions. If anything, just to speak with love in a soothing voice that shows emotional warmth. Through the eyes of a patient and an aspiring doctor, I visualize myself as a doctor who validates a patient's pain not as a statistic, but as an individual with peculiar interests, core values, and a unique life journey. Maybe one day, a little girl who comes to see me for her checkup would walk in with a smile. And nothing would make me happier than seeing that. •

Thought questions:
- Can a doctor be everything for everyone? If so, how? If not, why?
- Doctors have varying levels of emotional intelligence (EI). Should doctors be required to show proficiency in EI? Why or why not?
- What qualities of "best friendship" apply to the patient-doctor relationship and what are the differences between those types of relationships?

THE PERFECT DOCTOR

The View from the Other Chair

•

Miriam Colleran

The other chair is that extra one in the hospital outpatient room or at the inpatient bedside. Sometimes, it's plastic and functional. Other times, it's a high-backed, supportive, enveloping armchair. That chair can be uncomfortable. It's the seat for the family member, the carer.

My daughter has pulmonary capillaritis. It is a rare autoimmune disease that causes the lungs to bleed. Initially, she was diagnosed with pulmonary hemosiderosis. Both diseases cause bleeding in the person's lungs. The bleeds can vary from small to large and may cause shortness of breath, a dry cough or coughing up blood (hemoptysis). Untreated, the lungs may fibrose or harden in time. Treatment is aimed at either stopping a bleed or preventing long-term hardening of the lungs. As a physician-mom and carer, I sit in that other chair too frequently. It has been an unwanted opportunity to learn about being a doctor.

Entering the world of living with a serious illness is like living in a gated city. It can be an isolating and fearful place. Hidden within those fortified walls, patients and their loved ones need a haven to speak, to be listened to and to be heard. There is a need for physicians who are prepared to work with and accompany people living with serious illnesses, who will attend to them along the path. In that therapeutic space, a restorative patient and doctor dyad can form, transform and heal. Patients need doctors practicing compassionate care that is embedded in evidence informed clinical practice. For de-identification purposes, I will refer to all doctors by the pronoun "they."

When my daughter was two years old, she became pale and developed fatigue. Her bloodwork revealed an extreme anemia. The doctor was clear and purposeful as they explained by phone that the plan was to go to the emergency room of our local hospital urgently. She had a blood transfusion and was commenced on iron supplementation.

Shortly after the discontinuation of iron, she became anemic again and iron medication was restarted. The following month, she became very unwell and was breathing very rapidly. In the emergency department, there were shadows on her chest x-ray. These shadows indicated illness in the lungs but not the exact cause. They often indicate infection but, unbeknownst to us at the time, those shadows were hiding bleeding in her lungs.

Her oxygen saturations (the measurements of her blood oxygen by a probe usually on a finger) were repeatedly reading extremely low. Not long afterwards, a more senior doctor quietly and unobtrusively entered the room. They were knowledgeable and their therapeutic presence was calmly reassuring, consoling and capable. My daughter was commenced on intravenous antibiotics. The following evening, there was another conversation, but this time with a different physician. Their skillful communication made transferring a little girl of under three to intensive care to prevent her from tiring seem less daunting and logical. She had another blood transfusion, oxygen and intravenous antibiotics. She recovered as the doctor had predicted.

The following few years were times of greater calm. Then the disease uncovered itself again when she had her first episode of hemoptysis. Again, she got better after antibiotics. A month later, my daughter was playing in another outpatient room as I sat opposite our newest doctor for the first time. They listened attentively and patiently, occasionally interjecting with short, clarifying questions. While the physician's answers were brief and concise, they were truthful and helpful, and they showed understanding. There was no false hope nor evasion. It was clear to me that my daughter had an undiagnosed, serious illness.

So, I asked them, "What does she have?"

They replied, "Pulmonary hemosiderosis."

They discussed the plan for further investigations, a scan of her chest and a biopsy of her lung, to test for her disease. So, we left that office with a potential diagnosis and a plan of care from the doctor.

A few weeks later, this doctor came to our daughter's small hospital room to meet with us about the results of her biopsy (the sample of her lung tissue that was analyzed in a laboratory). My daughter had become very unwell after the bronchoscopy and open lung biopsy. The surgery which had provoked a sudden bleed in that lung. She was also in pain from the chest drain (a tube going into her chest) and the doctor said that they would return to meet with us. The unspoken message was that they wanted to meet in a different room and not at my five-year-old daughter's bedside. As a palliative care physician, I recognized all the signs of breaking bad news. A short while later, we sat at the table with the doctor and the accompanying nurse in a small sparse room. The physician appeared calm and unhurried. They explained that the biopsy confirmed that my daughter had pulmonary capillaritis. Their understated but effective leadership skills at the helm of the meeting were inclusive as they gently guided us at the start of an uncertain illness journey.

Sitting in the other chair, I have met many physicians in my role as her mother and carer. It is difficult to discuss disappointing experiences that have occurred. A chair, no matter how cozy, was comfortless in easing these experiences of disregard, disbelief, and sometimes kind dismissiveness. The fundamental ingredients in supportive therapeutic relationships were collaboration, compassion, humanity and sometimes humor, responsiveness, rapport, and 'therapeutic presence' (Widera & Smith, 2020). Knowledgeable, open-minded, human, humane and humble doctors helped to create a safe and easy space to engage with them.

Patients as people have differing needs at different times. Negotiating serious illnesses remains challenging. Sitting in the other chair may still be a worrying time for the family member or loved one. But the needed doctor, one who is compassionate, competent and kind, will help support both the patients and their loved ones through the walled city of the illness journey. •

Thought questions:
- How would you like to be treated if you were sitting in 'the other chair?'
- Should patients and caregivers who are physicians be treated any differently than other patients? If so, how?
- What are the different needs of caregivers to patients with acute illnesses versus chronic diseases? Should medical providers talk to these caregivers differently? If so, how?

Practice Your Humanity

•

Rohan Bhat

Taking care of others is a skill that is honed. Like any other skill, clinical acumen is impacted equally by experience and the effort one puts in. I have found in my clinical training that the physicians I admire most do not just have great clinical acumen, but they combine it with a bedside manner that forges therapeutic patient relationships. Despite any amount of accumulated clinical experience, guidelines for clinical practice are in a constant state of evolution. Can we as doctors promise to know every Uptodate article or each relevant professional society guideline at any given moment for our patients? For the vast majority, the answer is no. Can we work to refine our role as healers by combining our communication skills, ability to convey empathy, and ability to provide guidance and emotional support for our fellow suffering human beings? We can certainly try. Though this combination may not be infallible, this is the realm of our profession in which humanity trumps science.

As a medical student, it can be difficult to remember this human element that will accompany each patient we are bound to take care of. Despite many learning encounters with standardized patients for whom we are taught to express empathy, the focus is on knowing the treatment of disease on paper and the buzzwords that will guide us to the correct answer of an exam question. While the human and factual sides of learning are synergistic, they don't always feel harmonious.

I have accompanied my dad to appointments with several different oncologists over the past few years. Some days, I have come out of the appointment in awe of the physician's care, and other days I have come out disappointed to see the emphasis on disease overshadow care for the human. As my dad has progressed through his cancer treatment, I have seen doctors introduce an assortment of treatment options and clinical trial consent forms to consider and leave him to choose a path forward. Despite my dad's PhD in a scientific field and his intent to scientifically understand any diagnosis or drug his doctors present, sorting through all this information is stressful, particularly if it isn't accompanied by guidance that accounts for his wishes. As different medical therapies fail to produce a response and the side effect burden becomes more pronounced, I find myself hoping doctors will consider asking him what he hopes to achieve through his treatment and care. I hope for more care that places my dad and his wishes at the center of the decision algorithm. I am ever grateful for my dad's doctors who can outline every possible treatment option. Without hesitation, I would choose the one who asks him what is most important to him on this journey.

Knowing that one day I will be responsible for caring for patients along with their disease, my dad's varied experiences remind me that making a patient feel heard, understood, and cared for are what I want to make central to my practice. These abilities feel like a prerequisite for our role as healers. For much of the next year of my training, my competence and abilities will be judged not just by the medical facts I can remember and regurgitate, but also by whether I can listen to patients, empathize with them, and make them feel cared and advocated for. Keeping in mind my dad's care and treatment during my medical training has shifted my perspective. As I begin caring for patients on the wards this year, digesting their daily lab data and developing plans for each of their problems, I try to look at the big picture of how my team is healing a patient in their entirety. This does not always come naturally to me, but I am working to train my mind to put the patient before the disease.

These days, I am thrilled if my attending physician tells me they are impressed by my bedside manner and the relationships I forge with my patients. I value this more than the attending who evaluates me on whether I know the answers to every question they pose while we round. I have also come to recognize how deeply I must understand a concept to be able to thoroughly explain it to a patient, answer the questions they will have, and reassure them in the face of their concerns. To me, this illustrates the requisite blend of science and humanity in medicine. I have a growing appreciation for the inextricable human element of medicine, and I value the weight of my relationships with my patients. As I continue my training, I will remind myself that while knowing the science may help master one aspect of this profession, the physician-patient relationship is at the root of healing. •

Thought questions:
- Would you rather your doctor knew all the guidelines or treated you as a whole patient?
- Can empathy be taught?
- Is it ethical to offer chemotherapy to patients before asking their overarching wishes? Alternatively, is it ethical to hold lifesaving treatment that is against a patient's wishes?

Diversity and Ethics

•

making room for
all kinds of perfect

DIVERSITY AND ETHICS

A Neurologist Takes Paternity Leave

•

Vincent LaBarbera

As a parent to a newborn, I am perpetually in awe of my child. As a neurologist, I can't help but visualize nervous system myelination happening in real time. As she progresses through her infantile milestones, I am fortunate to be able to take time off from my medical practice. In making these observations (and constantly reminding myself and others to "support the neck!"), I also find I have some time to contemplate my life, professionally and personally. In taking this time, I see that parenthood and physician-hood share key characteristics. For me, these two supreme self-identities at times reflect one another, at times run seamlessly, and at other times pull in opposite directions. Ultimately, in my quest to be a better father, I also see a parallel mission to be a better physician.

Early in my medical school training, we learned about the pillars of medical ethics, upon which I have attempted to build my personal philosophy to care for patients. And in this way, I strive for perfection in my work—and conversely, I look back at that time (pre-children) and see that the same pillars also served as a foundation for trying to be the perfect parent.

Beneficence

Although non-maleficence, or more eloquently put *primum non nocere* ('first do no harm'), is the Hippocratic "first," I believe that at the very core of this profession is the desire to do good for others. All the best physicians I have known were not necessarily the fonts of encyclopedic knowledge, but instead projected an aura of considering the patients' best interests first. Even though physicians are often self-selected do-gooders, practicing beneficence is sometimes easier said than done. Thankfully, it can be learned and perfected through practice and mentorship. I've observed this in small and large ways in mentors during interactions with patients. They make little notes in a patient's chart remembering his partner's name, or that her favorite pastime is hiking. They make sure scripts are filled or prior authorizations are done in a timely manner. They visit a patient who is hospitalized for an unrelated issue. After a long clinic session, they call patients with results personally when follow up questions are anticipated. I also believe inherent to "doing good" for the patient is being present during the patient encounter. I think that patients sense when their physician is actively trying to do good by them, instead of simply clicking through lists on the computer screen.

I draw the parenting parallel here. I make sure that those who depend on me know that I'm on their team. I am learning (and re-learning every day) that my young children do better when they see me do better. My four-year-old reminds me that I need to help clean up my own mess after I left my dinner plate out (imitating what I told him to do a few hours before at lunchtime) and serves as a testament that I should always strive to keep my physical (and metaphorical) house in order. By "doing good," I can assist those I am caring for in reaching their best possible outcome.

Non-maleficence

It is easy enough to appreciate why the physician (or parent) should not do things to actively harm those under his or her care. However, sometimes in clinical practice, I have to actively remind myself that medications, procedures, or tests may have unintended risks or harms. The best doctors, whom I try to emulate, build non-maleficence into their everyday practice, and do so as a second nature.

Early on in my training, I staffed a case of a young teenager presenting with a new headache with an attending pediatric neurologist, who probably had more years of clinical experience than I had of being alive. No red flag features were present, the history was consistent with a migraine, and with the exception of some parental anxiety (which, in my pre-fatherhood days, I may have felt was excessive), the patient was, overall, appearing fairly well. I had suggested getting an MRI of the patient's brain "for further evaluation" (translating to "due to my inexperience, we should rule out *something, anything* causing the headache"). This elder statesman of the department, however, posited back to me, "What is the risk of getting an MRI?" I confidently mentioned, "There is no risk!", almost as if a billboard exclaiming "NO RADIATION = NO RISK" was projecting from my own head.

This attending then said, "But if there are no red flag features, the examination and ocular fundus exam is normal, and this is ultimately a benign migraine, this patient has the risk of getting in the car and getting into an accident on the way to the imaging center, or we run the risk of causing the patient and parent weeks of stress awaiting the test." This interaction has guided my medical decision making many times, when re-orienting myself to the phrase "first do no harm."

I see beneficence and non-maleficence as two sides of the same coin. However, in my perception of parenthood, these two can at times be at odds. It would be very easy to let my kids eat ice cream and chips every day to make them happy, but that would certainly be doing harm. Sticking to the "first do no harm" rule can feel paternalistic, and it may run counter to the next pillar.

Autonomy

There have definitely been times, in my experiences as a father to young children, when paternalism (defined by the Oxford dictionary as "the practice on the part of people in positions of authority of restricting the freedom and responsibilities of those subordinate to them in the subordinates' supposed best interest") is necessary. As exemplified above, I would be doing my kids a grave disservice if I let them live to their own childhood devices and eat ice cream all day.

However, this paternalistic tendency must be dissociated when working with people under your care as a physician. The physician should do his or her best to share in the patient's understanding and perception of the situation, giving precedence to the patient's desires, and ultimately to their consent. Medical students were surveyed about the most desirable physician qualities by Hurwitz et al. in 2013. They found that empathy was the most important physician characteristic (Hurwitz, 2013). Putting aside the concept of "selective paternalism," when instances of shared decision making break down in an emergency (Drolet, 2017), the best physicians I have seen provide patients with the facts, the options, and a recommendation, followed by time and support to make their decision.

Justice

I've found the final pillar to be most tricky in clinical care. It subsumes various concepts such as fair and equitable distribution of resources, value of care, and legality, among others. Particularly during the COVID pandemic, where rationing of care, especially ICU beds, was a looming reality, the concept of justice in organizing and apportioning care was ever-present. Thankfully, I did not have to directly deny anyone a hospital bed who required it. At times, I did have to allocate care by helping to manage the limited electroencephalogram machines in our hospital, or by providing different levels of care, such as seeing patients using telehealth, to COVID-vulnerable people in the clinic, and I had to balance human and technological resources in our electromyography laboratory. I observed doctors juggling these various resource limitations without compromising the integrity of their medical decision-making, which was very admirable to see.

At home, however, the justice of allocating resources was more difficult for me. My father, also a physician, and someone whose practice I've come to realize I had been emulating my entire life, always used to quip that being a physician was more of a vocation than a profession. I still hold that statement to be true, and it is one of my guiding principles that pushes me forward during those difficult patient interactions or long work hours. However, in taking my parental leave, I also realized that I was having a hard time "leaving" the practice. Although I had coverage, I couldn't shake the feeling that I was abandoning my patients. It took a lot of introspection and guidance from those closest to me to realize that equally as important (if not more so) were the needs of my growing family—they also needed me there. It was not "just" for my young children to often take second place to my concerns at work, such as staying late finishing notes and coming home after the kids were already in bed, or reviewing documents for tomorrow's cases instead of playing with my kids.

I believe that the internal angst that I felt, of not missing something with my patients, or of making doubly sure my patients were covered, will always drive me to try and be a better doctor to my patients, but I've come to realize that being a better parent is integral for my sense of personal wellness, integral for the happiness and growth of my family. This must take a high priority in order for me to function at my highest level when I am actually with patients. I have to believe that prioritizing my family when I am at home also will drive better patient outcomes; placing a higher value on one's family's well-being has been a major source of burnout prevention (Garcia, 2019). This intangible way of prioritizing my family when I am at home leads to tangible outcomes, such as an increase in time playing with my kids instead of typing patient notes; more stories read, instead of reading Epic; and more contentedness during my time away from medicine, instead of anxiety about the next (sometimes hypothetical) patient encounter. Because of these improvements at home, I have found that I can approach my patient visits with clarity and focus, utilizing my time in front of the patient more fruitfully.

I recognize that this essay runs the risk of making it seem that patients are equated, or relegated, to the likes of young children. Instead, my goal was to communicate that the "perfect doctor" and the "perfect parent" may not always be perfect. Instead, they hold those under their care in the highest esteem and seek the betterment of themselves in order to better care for those around them. •

Thought questions:
- As the author describes, sometimes beneficence towards family or patient care takes away from the capacity for beneficence towards the other. Could you describe how you have found or strive to find a balance between the two?
- When is selective paternalism in medicine acceptable in your view? For further reading on this topic, please refer to Drolet et al. (2017).
- What forces are at play that lead providers to order tests that aren't entirely necessary "just to be sure?" Does the section on non-maleficence in this piece change your perspective on this category of diagnostic testing?

Why I Want My Next Doctor to be a Foreign Medical Graduate

Robert Lamb

The following two pieces are different perspectives on the same physician's life story—one by the physician herself and one by her husband. Both offer unique glimpses into a pervasive problem affecting diversity in medicine.

The streets of Portoviejo, a small coastal town in Ecuador, are dusty, hot, and loud. In the summertime, it feels like the intense tropical sun is melting the pavement and everything that stands on it. This heat provides the perfect contrast for an ice cream sandwich (literally a piece of bread folded around a scoop of ice cream), or a tangy, salted bag of freshly cut green mangoes. It was on these streets that I first met Mayra. The daughter of a neurologist and a pediatric surgeon, you could have bet on Mayra becoming a doctor from the moment she was born. Even as she skipped down these hot and dusty streets as a young girl, dodging rickshaw drivers and honking taxis, her sights were always set on a higher ideal: that one day she would be a physician like her parents.

Mayra's journey took her from the modest confines of the Cristo Rey Catholic school next to the Portoviejo cemetery to the Universidad San Francisco de Quito, where she went to one of the most prestigious medical schools in the country. Growing up in Portoviejo however, she faced many barriers to becoming a doctor. Some of these were cultural: few women entered medical school in Ecuador, and even fewer graduated. Many (including female role models in Mayra's family) became pregnant during the long training period and abandoned their profession to raise children. Once Mayra began her medical school training in the capital city of Quito, there was also the stigma of being "de provincia": Coming from a smaller province like Manabi (where Portoviejo is the capital) meant you were at a disadvantage relative to the children of well-to-do Quiteño families. Many of Mayra's classmates from the capital already had international medical experience, had received extracurricular tutoring in English, science and math, and since long ago had been groomed to become a doctor.

Even so, Mayra excelled in medical school and eventually graduated at the top of her class. Once doctors finish medical school, most go on to do a multi-year residency program to sub-specialize in a specific field of medicine. Mayra could count on one hand the number of female neurologists she knew, but that only strengthened her conviction that she wanted to become a neurologist like her father. While there were several medical schools in the country and even a few residency programs, there was no residency available in Ecuador for neurology. That meant that Mayra not only had to overcome the gender bias in representation in the medical profession and her disadvantage coming from a coastal province in Ecuador, but she also had to compete with local and foreign medical graduates alike in pursuing medical residency in another country.

This point in Mayra's journey took her to the United States, where she studied for six months to take the U.S. medical licensing exams (USMLE). The USMLE is one of the most difficult tests in the world: It consists of four different sections, each one lasting up to nine hours, and covers basic anatomy and physiology, all of general medicine, patient care, and patient interaction. U.S. medical students are trained to pass each step of the USMLE as they go through medical school. Foreign medical graduates have to take the same exams, but they also have to overcome disadvantages of language, exam-specific preparation in school, and extra-curricular training. In addition, foreigners by default have historically had to score approximately 5% higher than U.S. medical graduates to be competitive for the same residency spot (NRMP, 2020). Worryingly, this may become even harder, since Step 1 of the USMLE was recently changed from a point score to a pass/fail score. This overwhelmingly places more focus on the medical school from which the applicant graduated, along with U.S.-based experience, all of which disfavors foreign medical graduates (Makhoul, 2020). Regardless, maybe one in a hundred students from other countries who start the journey to become a doctor in the United States actually make it. Mayra was one of them, and I can say with assurance she was one of the best.

After the USMLE, Mayra went to neurology residency at Brown University, an elite Ivy League school, and finished her training with a fellowship at the peak of the medical mountaintop: the Mayo Clinic in Minnesota. And yet despite her repeated successes, she is often seen by many patients and even colleagues as underqualified: a young, female, 5'3" Latin-American immigrant who has no business operating at the highest level of patient care and responsibility. Mayra has patients refer to her almost daily as "nurse," "honey," and "sweety." She has had patient family members ask when the real doctor is going to arrive, if they can see a male doctor, an older doctor, and someone with more experience. And always, Mayra continued to provide the utmost excellence in care. None of their complaints or doubts were based on facts; they simply couldn't see past what they assumed were deficiencies. I ask, if she is not the perfect doctor, who is?

DIVERSITY AND ETHICS

Foreign medical graduates constitute a critical component of our health system. For instance, 41% of all primary care physicians in the U.S. are from another country (Akl, 2007). Many foreign medical graduates take training positions and jobs in locations, medical fields, and hospital systems where U.S. doctors do not want to work for various reasons. As such they fill essential gaps in medical access, disproportionately working in high-need rural and urban areas (Goodfellow, 2016). And the representation of foreign medical graduates in the U.S. medical system is on the rise, having increased from 6.3% in 1959 to 14% in 1989, 23% in 1994, and 28% in 2006 (Woods, 2006).

Unrealistic expectations always exist in the medical field. Patients and their families are already under a great deal of stress when seeking care, causing tensions to run high and patience to run low. It is completely understandable to hope for and expect the best possible level of care. It's also important to recognize that the best possible care can look very different from expectations.

The next time I have to go see the doctor, I hope that it's a foreign medical graduate like Mayra who treats me. I know that they have been through the gauntlet ten times over just to be able to make it to where they are. I know that they have had to be better than the rest at every step, overcoming bias and excelling beyond a shadow of a doubt in order to receive the respect and acceptance of their peers. This is the perfect doctor for me. •

Thought questions:
- Would Mayra have been different as a physician had she trained in the United States? If so, how?
- Being called pet names by patients or facing assumptions that someone is not the doctor because of the way they look are types of micro-aggressions. The Oxford Dictionary defines micro-aggressions as "indirect, subtle, or unintentional discrimination against members of a marginalized group." Have you ever experienced micro-aggressions? Describe how they made you feel. What are some techniques to face and cope with micro-aggressions?
- Do you have implicit bias against doctors or medical providers based on gender, race, ethnicity, appearance, training background, or other qualities? If so, describe your bias, think about its origin, and think of three ways to curb it. Strategies include awareness, acceptance, getting to know people with qualities you may fear or misunderstand, and imagining yourself in their shoes. There are many resources online to learn more about implicit bias and its impact on health care, including the U.S. Department of Health and Human Services Office of Minority Health, the Kirwan Institute for the Study of Race and Ethnicity at Ohio State University, and outsmartingimplicitbias.org.

THE PERFECT DOCTOR

A Good Doctor

•

Mayra Montalvo

I was born to be a neurologist.
I am from Ecuador. There is no neurology residency in Ecuador.

The beginnings are never easy. We moved to Barcelona while my parents did their medical residency when I was four years old. I had to skip a grade due to the different education schedule. I did not know the letters while everyone else in class did, but by the end of the year I was the top student, and the teachers asked my dad to buy me a list of books because I had finished all the ones they had to offer me in class. This wasn't even in my native Spanish, but in Catalan.

After four years, we went back to my hometown of Portoviejo with dusty streets, back to my now unfamiliar Spanish with a different accent and a different culture. I was the best student in high school, but that was more a testament to the low education standards in my part of the world than to any effort on my part. I went to study medicine in Quito, the big city where I found myself now competing against a well-trained, incredibly talented and intelligent cohort of would-be doctors. I knew from day one that the big-city high schools had prepared the other students better. I got a D on my first chemistry test and had to drop calculus so I could take precalculus since I had no knowledge of these things. I was also the target of racist prejudice and sexualization since I was from the coastal province of Manabi. I was the "mona," the monkey. Many people called me that with affection, but I was never given the chance to simply be another medical student. I adapted, I learned, and I eventually graduated top of my class.

Then came a grueling three-year process of volunteering in clinics, job shadowing, working as a research assistant, studying for exams, and taking the arduous U.S. medical licensing exam. I was fortunate to get a score high enough to land a neurology residency at an Ivy League university. Many, if not most, of the cohort I studied with for the exams were not so lucky. One man my age (we are all doctors already at this point) threw up in the middle of the first exam due to his nerves.

I remember my father always said when I was a child, "There is nothing harder or more grueling than residency." I thought getting into a prestigious medical residency coming from a developing country was a challenge. But residency is different. Residency years are like dog years, because each year counts as seven. Because you live life so intensely, learn so much in so little time and work three times more while sleeping twice as little as what a normal person should. All this is on top of always having to be at peak performance because you don't want your lack of knowledge and sleep to hurt a patient. Multiple times, my co-residents and I would cry in the stairwell, feeling as if we were giving our everything but still somehow that was not enough.

It got a little easier during fellowship, but the demeaning and discriminatory comments did not disappear. I love neurology, I love the cases, I love the anatomy, I love the challenge, I love my patients and care deeply for their families. But, sometimes I am the victim of vicious, undeserved hate from these same people. It's hard to survive this gauntlet. It's harder still to be a really good physician, and when your patient's adult daughter refuses to let you provide potentially life-saving treatment because you didn't graduate from a U.S. medical school, it deflates your instinct to help. Of course, the attending on staff at the time, a Black woman, also wasn't good enough because she had gone to a state school.

After the altercation, the attending and I shared a look that said it all. We didn't need to bring up the obvious stigma we were both facing on a daily basis. Another patient told me that he did not understand how someone from a third world country could be practicing in one of the best hospitals in the world. He meant it as a compliment, but the comment still stings.

Throughout my life, I have had to deal with patients and coworkers alike who paint a version of me in their heads long before the quality of my work can speak for itself. How can you be a top physician if you are a young, pretty woman from Latin America, with an accent and a bright smile? Discrimination against health care providers undermines our ability to do our jobs and does a number on self-esteem. Understand that your doctor will not always be the classic white male portrayed to you in so many books, movies and TV shows. Good doctors come in different shapes and colors. See beyond stereotypes. Let diversity make us stronger. •

Thought questions:
- Has anyone ever refused your help because of the way you looked? If not, have you ever witnessed discrimination? What are some strategies to cope with such experiences for both the victim and bystander?
- Put yourself in the shoes of the patient's daughter who refused care from Dr. Montalvo and her attending. What do you imagine was going through her mind?
- Whose responsibility is it to curb discrimination? Should hospitals have zero tolerance policies for discrimination against staff and providers?
- How has an interpersonal challenge made you stronger? How did you respond, how do you wish you had responded, and how will you respond next time?

The Best Doctors Stay Awake

Melissa Flanagan

The speakerphone at the center of the table blasted Haitian-Creole, the interpreter's voice toggling between me, the treating psychiatrist, and a desperate wife and mother just as fearful at the thought of her husband coming home as she was of hearing the reasons why he likely could not. From across the table, I told her about the New York State psychiatric hospital system and its paucity of options, and I listened to her concerns for the man who was well when they married. The psychiatrist seated next to me had been tasked with discussing treatment and prognosis, until I turned my head to address him and discovered: He was asleep.

Beautiful dreamer, chin-on-chest, glasses sliding lower and lower, down past my expectation that to be the kind of doctor who comforts and connects with the poor, the disempowered, the traumatized and the terrorized, one must start by staying awake. I don't remember how I woke him. I'm sure I dissociated from the horror; I might have used my elbow. I wanted to use an air horn.

There she was, a working class Haitian immigrant, a woman of color, sole provider for a family whose lives were falling apart on that ward, while she watched an affluent, educated man sleep, someone who held the details of her pain and the power to medicate, to legally commit, to label, and to decide whether her husband would go home to restart a cycle of aggression and re-hospitalization, or whether he would go away to receive long-term care, which would make her 100 percent responsible for running a household well below the poverty line. The gravity of her crisis was lost to the dreams of a man so disaffected by her that he fell asleep. It was an unintentional, albeit devastating, power move.

The physician-social worker collaboration in health care settings is a dysfunctional, arranged marriage of two people often from completely different villages. We usually come together out of necessity and not because we share training experiences, parallel worldviews, or similar socioeconomic realities. The income disparity alone aligns a social worker more closely with the way most patients, and most people, live, and informs a more pragmatic assessment of person-in-environment that is critical to treating the whole patient realistically. We are trained to approach people and systems through a social justice paradigm, which means we look for racial biases, economic disparities, and power differentials, many of which fester on our own treatment teams.

One afternoon, a hospital attending who sat on a committee with me returned from his first run as a guest physician with a mobile mental health team, which had just visited a patient in his home. The doctor was animated, invigorated by the experience of traveling into the community to see where and how a city hospital patient lived. "The smells!" he told our group excitedly, "I had forgotten what an apartment building smelled like, I've lived in a house for so many years." I questioned how a man who had treated thousands of patients in a New York City public hospital had forgotten about apartment life, and I wondered how he felt confident in the care he provided without understanding the environments where his patients would manage and recover from their illnesses.

More than once, I have sent clients with multiple comorbidities, who were living in a homeless shelter, their scalps vibrating with scabies, to local emergency rooms for permethrin treatments and psychiatric evaluations related to unsafe self-care, only to have them immediately return. One night, a doctor called to tell me that my concern about a client in their ER was "a social problem and not a medical one," so he sent the client back to the shelter, with directions to cover her head and body with permethrin on her own, for several days, when self-neglect was a hallmark of her illness, at odds with her ability to adhere to complicated, multi-step directions in a bathroom and dorm room shared by other residents. Before the doctor hung up, he admonished me for expecting the hospital "to solve all the problems."

But then, one summer, a psychiatric unit chief asked me if our patient's home had air conditioning. My ears moved like sonar toward him. It was, on the surface, a seemingly innocuous data point, but a brilliant one that helped inform this doctor's algorithm of discharge readiness. His eyes were open to the necessity of understanding how his patients lived and the role of the environment in maintaining stability in the community. He envisioned our patient, a man with a history of violence and treatment non-adherence, who often visited his mother in her apartment, where he was known to sit naked in her living room. Whatever risk we calculated in sending him home would only worsen amid the claustrophobia, discomfort, and irritability brought on by the summer heat. Discharge readiness would look different for him, and for other patients, based on the temperature they would return to. It was next-level doctoring.

In the winter of 2021, my neurosurgeon sat a few inches across from me on a rolling stool in his office and said to me, "If you were my wife, I would want you to do this." With just five words, "if you were my wife," he reached across an epic power divide and helped me decide to have pipeline embolization surgery to fix an unruptured left ophthalmic segment brain aneurysm that appeared as an incidental finding on an MRI ordered for some vision problems I was concerned about. He calculated my risk factors for a rupture across the rest of my lifespan, with an understanding of my role as a wife and a parent of a young child. He considered how I lived and what I didn't want to lose. He drew parallels between his own wife and me, similar in age, and with shared expectations of the future. His surgical acumen carried me through the procedure, but his humanity was the prelude to resolving my ambivalence and preserving the future I envisioned.

The magic in medicine lies here, at a place that feels personal and humble, where there is self-awareness of privilege and class, respect for air conditioners, and the fierce protection of someone else's wife. It is a commitment to wakefulness in the face of a stranger's pain. •

Thought questions:
- How can doctors become more aware of social determinants of health?
- Whose responsibility is it to instill "respect for air conditioners?" Is it that of the government? The educational system? Parents? Doctors? Medical educators? Hospital administration? Or, only social services?
- Brainstorm how attending to social determinants of health can be paid for. Is it the job of taxpayers, health insurance companies, employers, or others?

Fading Photographs and Mournful Memories: Reflections on the Humans Behind Medical Complications

•

Chinmayi Balusu

I remember brushing the dust off a silver photo frame on top of a bookshelf in my parent's house when I was in elementary school, standing on a chair to reach it. The pleasant smiles of two young women and a man met my eyes. I recognized my mother's (*Amma* in Telugu, my native language) and aunt's features, with the backdrop of my great-grandparent's garden in Gudlavalleru, the village in the southeastern Indian state of Andhra Pradesh that has been home to my family for generations. The third person is my uncle, Amma's younger brother who passed away in 2000. I never had a chance to meet him except through his photographs and the memories Amma shared.

Amma used to tell me that he had passed away after becoming sick, but the explanation became more complex over the years. In the end, I learned that he had died following complications from an abdominal surgery that was performed by a medical resident in training. My initial reaction was anger: one mistake cost the life of my then 28-year-old uncle. I had many questions come to mind. Was the medical resident reckless and overconfident? Were they more concerned with their own learning experience rather than my uncle's health? Was my uncle just another surgery scheduled for the operation theater that day?

Looking back, I realize that my anger was rooted in the assumption that the error was made out of egoism, influenced by my personal connection and emotional state at the moment. In reality, there could have been a number of factors that contributed to the mistake. Perhaps the medical resident did not have adequate supervision, felt unprepared when they were asked to step up to perform this procedure, or felt that they would face severe repercussions if they spoke up. It's easy for any of us to point fingers and place the blame. It is difficult to reconcile acceptance, forgiveness, empathy, anger, and grief when coming to terms with the fact that the doctors whom you place trust in to care for a loved one could inadvertently end up also harming them.

I revere the medical profession, yet I often wonder about these unseen patients' stories and lives that forever remain in the aftermath of medical errors, beyond the confines of statistical reports. Perhaps many of these stories are sidelined in medical trainees and professionals' pursuit of perfection and accuracy. I am not sure if the trainee doctor who performed the surgery on my uncle that day remembers him. I hope they do, and that they reflect on his case once in a while. Not from a point of never-ending self-guilt, but as a humanistic learning experience.

As I set out on my own medical journey, I jot down traits and core values that I would like to embody as a future physician: being grounded as an active listener, honestly acknowledging when I am not certain, and balancing the right amount of preventative caution. But it is inevitable that, even if I can refine all of these attributes, I might be involved in a medical error at some point over the course of my career, similar to that trainee. Someone might be in the same position as my uncle, and their family may experience the same grief.

In many cultural communities, including my own, doctors are often referred to as gods, with their medical skills and ability to save lives being equated with divine perfection. As a result, when medical errors occur and people are harmed, it can be difficult to reconcile the belief in doctors' god-like status with the reality. Even the most experienced and skilled doctors are still human, and mistakes can happen. Doctors may feel pressured to live up to this idealized image of perfection, leading to burnout and stress. It is important to acknowledge this reality and work towards creating a culture of communication—among doctors, patients, and their families—that encourages transparency, accountability, and learning from mistakes.

Achieving a sense of perfection in the aftermath of medical errors may look different for each individual involved. For some, a perfect closure may take the form of a formal apology from the medical institution or the individual responsible for the incident. For others, advocating for policy changes or reforms within the medical field to prevent similar errors from occurring in the future may be more meaningful. At the end of the day, there is no one-size-fits-all solution. What works for one family or doctor may not work for another.

Through advances in technology, sanitation practices, interprofessional collaborations, and beyond, the frequency of medical errors is decreasing overall (Rodziewicz et al, 2023). However, the experiences of family members who lose patients to medical errors remain constant and often invisible. While we cannot bring back patients who have lost their lives to medical error, both families and doctors can honor their memories by finding a mutual understanding, learning from the experience, and taking action to achieve their own sense of medical perfection that was absent before. •

DIVERSITY AND ETHICS

Thought questions:
- If you were the author's family, what would help you make peace with a potential medical error that may have caused their loved one's death?
- Have you heard of "second victim syndrome"? Second victims are defined as: "health care providers who are involved in an unanticipated adverse patient event, in a medical error and/or a patient related injury and become victimized in the sense that the provider is traumatized by the event. Frequently, these individuals feel personally responsible for the patient outcome. Many feel as though they have failed the patient, second guessing their clinical skills and knowledge base." (Scott, 2009) Have you ever experienced or witnessed someone experiencing second victim syndrome? What advice would you give to them?
- How should medical systems respond to medical errors? Should there be punishment for lack of remorse after a medical error?
- Will artificial intelligence increase or decrease the rates of medical errors?

For more information on medical errors, please refer to the Institute of Medicine's report *To Err is Human: Building a Safer Health System.*

THE PERFECT DOCTOR

Immigrating Into Medicine

•

Pouya Ameli

The very word "professionalism" conjures emotionally charged memories. Too often, it's code for: "We'd like for you to walk, talk, and dress in a manner that fits *our* traditions."

When my family emigrated from Iran to the U.S., we clung to the ideals that had served our ancestors, the ideals that served us, the ideals that brought us together in our new environment teeming with challenges. Growing up in a gang-ridden neighborhood, my family endured by clinging to those principles. Those solid roots allowed me to go from hearing gunshots in the middle of the night to donning a white coat. I remember standing in line at a convenience store with my mother. I caught a glimpse of the display of candies and chocolates. As I drew closer to gaze at the options, suddenly, an elderly white man with a war veteran cap yelled, "Hey! Don't touch that. Take your disease back to where you came from!" I ran back to my mother. Later, I'd learn that my mother wanted to respond, but remained silent when the cashier whispered, "He's old. Just leave him alone." Despite the kindness of the cashier, I have never forgotten the fear and anger that moment created. I never expected to have feelings like that in medicine, where I thought I would be welcomed for my unique qualities.

When you apply to medical school, there is so much emphasis on diversity. Yet the traditional definitions of success many of us hold so dear often do not allow for divergence of mindset and behavior. Admit it, there's an archetype of success in medicine—not just the knowledge and quality of patient care, but the way doctors carry themselves, the way they speak, the way they look. How much of that is truly necessary to be successful, and how much is a vestige of our past? It sometimes feels like we're systematically disincentivizing the very diversity that supposedly strengthens us.

My mother frequently told me stories about my Persian heritage. She painted pictures of Persian contributions to the world—their inventions and innovations. I didn't always realize how much my parents sacrificed to give me the opportunities I have in the United States. To open doors for me, they closed doors on an established life of comfort and relative wealth in a country that housed their families and many of their most cherished memories. As I grew older, I began to realize what they had done and I demanded more and more of myself—not just for my benefit, but to make their sacrifice worth it. At times, my ambition outpaced my abilities and I paid the price. I have yet to find the words to accurately describe the breadth of emotions I feel when I think about the amazing feat that my parents were able to accomplish, so I'll keep it simple: My win is *our* win.

I graduated medical school, got married, and had children of my own. After hitting each milestone, I thought about what it would be like to drop everything, move to a different country, speak a different language, and start over. I imagine the immense stress one must feel when making such an anguishing decision like my parents did years ago.

However, despite the monumental meaning my achievements carry for my family, the truth about this career that I've spent so much time and energy pursuing is that advancement often means assimilating yourself into the culture of your environment, however unnatural it may feel. As a child, I learned about the importance of honesty, of saying the truth even when it's hard to say or hard to hear. In medicine, it's easy to be *too* honest. You have to be careful about what opinions, emotions, or experiences you share and often have to leave your "baggage" at the door. Even many of the most powerful people would frequently rather you be polite than be correct. Why is this? People are busy—they don't have the time or capacity to sit and learn about your view of the world. The demands are high and the time is limited. As a result, we default to long-established ways of being that leave no room for true diversity.

At times, I was bitter or angry about working so hard to enter a field where I often didn't feel valued or seen. But today, my soul is not crushed—in fact, it is alive and well. I've written my bildungsroman, at least in my own mind, where it really counts. My roots are strong and resilient. They've endured thousands of microaggressions, feelings of not belonging, periods of self-doubt, frustrations, and tears. I remember crying in the stairwells of my residency hospital, asking why I had chosen this path and searching for answers. I eventually found them.

I love medicine not just for what it has given me, but also what it has demanded from me. I'm not sure all the bad days were necessary, but I like who I am, so it's hard for me to be angry about the trials and tribulations that made me this way. Do I think it needed to be as hard as it was? No. Do I think it should have been easy? Also no. There is growth in the struggle, but when there is too much struggle, especially if it's not recognized—that's a problematic system.

As a physician, as a servant to society, as an advocate for the downtrodden, I want to pave the path for others like me. Sometimes, I campaign to have our struggles acknowledged. Sometimes, I reframe the path as one that was never meant to be easy to traverse. Always, I seek to unite people of varying backgrounds to understand that, at the end of the day, we're all humans pursuing happiness. •

Thought questions:
- Have you seen the field of medicine clash with individual cultural practices of doctors and health care workers? If so, describe how.
- Are there elements of the traditional culture of western medicine that should be left behind to make room for diversity? If so, which ones?
- Are there elements of diverse cultural practices that get in the way of professionalism? If so, which ones?
- The author writes that he does not think that medical training needed to be as hard as it was for him, nor does he think it should be easy. What are the necessary difficulties of medical training and what are unnecessary difficulties? How should medical education change to minimize unnecessary difficulties?

DIVERSITY AND ETHICS

Medicine Blinders

•

Alejandra Casillas

On one clinic day, I was introduced to Mrs. A, one of our patients at a federally qualified health center in West Los Angeles, where I supervise medical students and residents during their clinical rotations in internal medicine. Mrs. A appeared nervous as the resident and I walked her through the steps of working up her abnormal mammogram with subsequent studies, and perhaps a biopsy. An abnormal mammogram marked her first entry into health care after going many years without medical services. She had been living with no immigration documentation which had limited her access to primary care, and it had been challenging to know where to get non-emergency care. Now in her late 50s, and with her life more stable from a social perspective, she was beginning to receive regular medical services at our free clinic.

We delineated the findings and the process in Spanish, Mrs. A's native language. The very capable and fantastic resident had already briefed me on our patient before I came in the room—she had a sense that Mrs. A was hesitant about proceeding. Was she confused by the medical jargon? Was she anxious about talking about the possibility of cancer? Mrs. A had not said much, but she was teary-eyed. As I walked in the clinic room, I prepared to put on my "Latina daughter" hat, in addition to my white coat. My first instinct was that she simply needed more information to be distilled in a way that was not so intimidating. Perhaps she needed the complicated facts to be explained by me in a way that felt familiar and comfortable—much like how I would approach such a conversation about following up on important test results with my own Spanish-speaking mother.

But despite my back and forth with Mrs. A, we were not making much headway. I was not sure that Mrs. A would leave our visit today with an intent to proceed with our recommendations.

"*Okay, Señora A, hacemos una cita para la próxima semana y usted nos dice que decide.* Okay, Mrs. A., we will make a visit for next week, and you can let us know what you decide."

As I proceeded to start to end the visit, I told myself that we did what we could. Time was precious and clinic was busy. The resident was already racing on to the next patient. I wrapped up the consult and my hand started to reach for the doorknob.

"*Pero doctora, le puedo preguntar algo?* But doctor, can I just ask you something?"

I said, "Yes..."

Mrs A. continued in Spanish. "What about what they are saying, what they are saying about the president on TV. If I keep using this clinic, will they take away my green card application? My neighbor said I should just stop coming here. I saw it on the news. How can I do all these tests? What do you think I should do?"

My heart sank. The medicine blinders lifted.

Yes, the medicine blinders. Let me explain. When horses race on a racetrack, they actually have "blinders" placed on them. Racers cover up the horses' eyes laterally to prevent peripheral "distractions." It makes the racehorses oblivious to anything but the racetrack. It forces them to have tunnel vision. It is almost as if they are in their own little world. To go faster. To be "better."

My medicine blinders had left me blind to my patient's cry for help.

At the time of this patient visit, in the fall of 2017, the Trump administration had started publicizing a proposed policy change in which an immigrant holding a visa could be passed over for getting permanent residency—a green card—if they use Medicaid, a subsidized ACA plan, or a list of other government benefits.

I remember seeing this come up in the news and had even discussed it with my own family. We dismissed it as hyped-up rumors to dissuade people from receiving needed care. I thought it was impossible nonsense. But was it possible? At the time, I didn't really know.

As I looked at Mrs. A to answer, my heart sank again further, and I prepared to give an unsatisfying response.

I told her that I didn't think this was possible. But I also didn't have definitive answers or guarantees about this. Yes, she had Medicaid and she was in the process of applying for her green card. But receiving her green card would be of *no* use, if she was not around to use it. Her health would have to come first above all things. Her kids needed her now. She needed this medical work-up to stay healthy and keep moving forward.

"*Es todo lo que le puedo decir, pero se que todo esto es muy difícil.* That is all I can tell you, but I know that this is all very difficult," I said to Mrs. A. She nodded in acceptance and stated she would make arrangements for her follow up tests with our coordinator.

It should have felt like a "win." But the irony of this conversation was not lost on me. I am the daughter of two formerly undocumented immigrants. I am the cousin of undocumented mothers and fathers. I know what it is like to constantly live with this fear. I remember feeling that sensation in the pit of my stomach—feeling afraid to ask for any help... and just needing to be invisible. Helping patients that live with these fears and these stigmas and getting them into care is a core part of who I am as a physician. It is why I went into medicine. And yet, I didn't recognize the fear inside Mrs A. How could I have not instantly seen it? Or at least have looked around, asked her, and delved deeper given her history on presentation?

Sometimes our practice of medicine can be like the horses on the racetrack. We walk into the patient room with blinders on in order to be able to take care of all the patients we need to take care of. However, being better in medicine actually requires us to be as fully sensitive to our patients' surroundings and context. Mrs. A reminded me I need to stay deeply connected with the humane and vulnerable parts of my past and present self in order to be the most in-tune and astute physician that I can be. That is what I uniquely bring to medicine. It is a fight every day to keep the medicine blinders from taking that away from me.

Thank you for that needed reminder, Mrs. A. *Gracias.* •

Thought questions:
- This story describes how "medicine blinders" can cause doctors to overlook important social aspects of patient care. How can blinders make doctors better? Who do they make doctors better for?
- When was a time when you have become aware of your own blinders? Who reminded you and how? What did you do with this new awareness?
- Are there any downsides to doctors taking their blinders off and being less focused on the racetrack? If so, what are they? How should doctors strike a balance between focus on their subject matter and awareness of social determinants of health?

THE PERFECT DOCTOR

Secret Weapon

•

Chidinma Onweni

She gowns up, puts her N95 mask on, eye shield on, and gloves on. She looks through the glass window and sees the patient and a woman sitting with a clipboard that held animal pictures in boxes, who nods her in.

She walks into the room and states, "Good morning!"

The patient responds, "Good morning."

The woman sitting with the clipboard states, "The trays are over there."

The doctor responds, "I am not here for the tray. I am the physician."

What does a doctor look like? I am far from perfect in any area including my personal life. Wait, I take that back. There is no differentiation between work life and personal life for me. Medicine is my life and the only life that seems to belong to me. So, it hurts deeply when I am not recognized for what I am. I can take the tray, but that is not what I came in to do. I came in to examine my patient, and maybe on my way out, I can take the tray too.

College shaped me to strive, and medical school was difficult as expected and not as expected. It was my first exposure to the struggles that come along with being a physician that looks and sounds like me. Residency and fellowship were very rewarding. I was so grateful, and focused on training and succeeding that any experience or situation that did not align with these goals was not noticed.

Now, being a full-time practicing physician has been difficult to say the least. I wish medicine or knowledge was the difficult part, but it is not. It is everything else. What are these other things? It is people not expecting me to be a physician. Biases. Overt dismissal. Feeling like I need to conform.

Her tone.

She is smart, but her questions make me feel small.

Every decision I make or suggest being questioned, but not the decision of the person standing beside me despite them having less evidence and facts. Believing the lies that I am less than. Imposter Syndrome. Feeling like a fraud for not passing my boards on the first try.

Three years into being an attending, it was time to take a step back and ask myself, what was the original reason or goal to pursue a career in medicine? The answer was to heal. As simple and as unsophisticated as that may sound, it is the truth. I wanted to be part of healing, part of the process that brings our fellow human beings back to health. I wanted to be a person who is assumed to be a doctor despite how she looks. A person who is admired by colleagues. A person who publishes articles and moves the specialty forward through contributions to research and inventions. I wanted to touch lives and apply the art of science.

The journey of becoming a physician involves giving up part of yourself, sometimes all of yourself. To that, I borrow the saying from John 15:13, "What manner of love is this that you lay your life down for a friend."

You give up your young adulthood days to study. You give up family time, friends, events, hobbies, and travel. You spend more years training and, when you start practicing, if you are not spending every minute thinking or doing something patient related, then you feel guilty. You feel like you are neglecting your patients. You have laid your life down for your friend, the patient. And if you had to do it all over again, you would do it with no hesitation.

In one episode of the show *The Rookie: Feds*, a Black woman FBI agent is sent in as an undercover paramedic with a real paramedic as her partner. The killer suspects that something is wrong and asks, "Why will they send two paramedics for a job one paramedic can do? One of you is the FBI!" He chose the white man as the fake paramedic FBI agent and presumed that the Black woman was the real paramedic. This was the wrong assumption. The FBI calls the Black woman their "secret weapon—no one sees her coming." No one expects her to be FBI because she is a Black woman. In that episode, the FBI won their fight because of their "secret weapon."

I hope to be my medical specialty's "secret weapon." Since no one expects me to be good, "no one will see me coming." •

Thought questions:
- Have you ever been treated differently because of how you looked? How did you, or how would you react?
- Is it doctors' responsibility to speak up when they are treated unfairly? Or is it the system's responsibility to be accepting of different types of doctors?
- Have you ever seen, faced or heard of repercussions for students and doctors speaking up for equity, especially within the hierarchy of medicine? What is the best way to handle these repercussions?

Afterword

Creating and telling stories is a uniquely human activity. The stories you have just read are special. They report the reflections of medical students, physicians and health care professionals as they experience the challenges that foster their development, learning and personal growth. Seminal experiences such as learning how to be with voluble patients, deciding to care for a patient and be late for a school event, learning to listen to the feedback of patients as much as the feedback of supervisors all are the times of growth that leaven the perfectionism so prevalent in medical students. Caring for a child or patient who dies is always memorable and powerful. Putting the event in words, poetry or prose enhances both the meaning and the richness of the memory. Other stories highlighted the impact of bias and the reality of being "other" through color, ethnicity or foreign birth and education, and the reality of personal experience of illness and the journey through burnout to self-care.

Reading these stories makes me reflect on my more than four-decade career as a pediatrician, child and adolescent psychiatrist and medical educator. I find myself thinking about dilemmas I have faced and especially the painful lessons I have learned. I have found the challenge of helping a patient manage harmful behaviors and self-destructive urges particularly poignant. I try to engage the patient in a partnership to alter behavior and create hope for a different way of soothing and living. I find myself feeling that controlling the patient's impulses is my responsibility, that I must be perfect at that and that I cannot fail.

Sarah was one of those patients for whom I felt responsible. She was adamant about being thin and extremely successful at losing weight. It became an obsession of hers. I was her psychiatrist and talked with her weekly for over three years. She enjoyed our talks and would tell me about her college courses and her classwork. She would share with me her freelance writing after graduation. We would make plans for her to eat more, but her weight would hover around 70 pounds. She looked ill but refused hospitalization. Previous inpatient stays had led to weight gain which she promptly lost after discharge. It was painful for me to see her and frustrating for me to not be able to help her change. Medication trials and consultations were uniformly fruitless.

Sarah died of chronic malnutrition at age 28, a victim of severe intractable anorexia nervosa. I stayed with her marveling at the books she authored, saddened by her untimely death and wondering what more I could have done for her.

In all of these stories, students and practitioners find the richness of the practice of medicine through relationships, shared journeys and an appreciation of one's humanness as a physician. Mistakes occur, we learn to listen and engage, and we come to value our privileged positions as professionals who use our knowledge, our skills and our values to understand, to witness, to care for and ultimately to love our patients. This development, growth and change is so vividly presented in these stories. We are richer for them; they are instructive for us all.

John Sargent, MD
Chief of Child and Adolescent Psychiatry, Professor
Tufts University School of Medicine •

References

•

Alda A. Does your doctor care about you? Clear+Vivid with Alan Alda. Published May 18, 2021. Accessed November 15, 2022. https://getpodcast.com/podcast/clearvividwithalanalda/does-your-doctor-care-about-you_29dab156c0.

Alpert JS, Frishman WH. The Most Important Qualities for the Good Doctor. Am J Med. 2021; 134(7): 825-826. doi:10.1016/j.amjmed.2020.11.002.

Akl EA, Mustafa R, Bdair F, Schünemann HJ. The United States physician workforce and international medical graduates: Trends and characteristics. J Gen Intern Med. 2007; 22: 264–268.

Barbieri A. 'Be interested, be curious, hear what's not said': how I learned to really listen to people. The Guardian. https://www.theguardian.com/lifeandstyle/2021/jul/24/interested-curious-how-i-learned-to-really-listen-to-people. Published July 24, 2021. Accessed November 13, 2022.

Branch WT, Pels RJ, Harper G, Calkins D, Forrow L, Mandell F, Maynard E, Peterson L, Arky RA. "A New Educational Approach for Supporting the Professional Development of Third-Year Medical Students." Journal of General Internal Medicine 1995; 10: 691-694.

Cameron RA, Mazer BL, DeLuca JM, Mohile SG, Epstein RM. In search of compassion: a new taxonomy of compassionate physician behaviours. Health Expect. 2015; 18(5): 1672-1685. doi:10.1111/hex.12160.

Coles R. The Call of Stories: Teaching and the Moral Imagination. Houghton-Mifflin; 1989.

Drolet BC, White CL. Selective paternalism. Virtual Mentor. 2012;14(7):582-588. Published July 1, 2012. doi:10.1001/virtualmentor.2012.14.7.oped2-1207.

Ely W. Every Deep Drawn Breath. New York, NY: Simon & Schuster, 2021.

Garcia CL, Abreu LC, Ramos JLS, et al. Influence of Burnout on Patient Safety: Systematic Review and Meta-Analysis. Medicina (Kaunas). 2019; 55(9): 553. Published August 30, 2019. doi:10.3390/medicina55090553.

Goodfellow A, Ulloa JG, Dowling PT, et al. Predictors of primary care physician practice location in underserved urban or rural areas in the United States: A systematic literature review. Acad Med. 2016; 91: 1313–1321.

Halpern J. What is Clinical Empathy? J Gen Intern Med. 2003; 18(8): 670-674. doi:10.1046/j.1525-1497.2003.21017.x.

Harper G. Breaking taboos and steadying the self in medical school. Lancet 1993; 342: 913-915.

Harper G. Epilogue. In Pories S, Jain S, Harper G, eds. The Soul of Medicine: Harvard Medical Students confront Life and Death. New York, NY: 2013, 2nd edition.

Hurwitz S, Kelly B, Powis D, Smyth R, Lewin T. The Desirable Qualities of Future Doctors—A Study of Medical Student Perceptions. Med Teach. 2013; 35(7): e1332-e1339. doi:10.3109/0142159X.2013.7701302.

REFERENCES

Kohn LT, Corrigan JM, Donaldson MS, eds. To Err is Human: Building a Safer Health System. Washington, DC: Committee on Quality of Health Care in America, Institute of Medicine. National Academies Press; 2000. ISBN: 9780309068376.

Lachman P. The Age of Kindness. ISQua. Published March 30, 2021. Accessed November 13, 2022. https://isqua.org/latest-blog/the-age-of-kindness.html.

Makhoul AT, Pontell ME, Ganesh Kumar N, Drolet BC. Objective Measures Needed—Program Directors' Perspectives on a Pass/Fail USMLE Step 1. N Engl J Med 2020 Jun 18; 382(25): 2389-2392.

National Academies of Sciences, Engineering, and Medicine, Committee on Systems Approaches to Improve Patient Care by Supporting Clinician Well-Being. (2019). Taking Action Against Clinician Burnout: A Systems Approach to Professional Well-Being. National Academies Press. Retrieved from https://nam.edu/systems-approaches-toimprove-patient-care-by-supporting-clinician-well-being.

National Resident Matching Program. Charting Outcomes in the Match: International Medical Graduates. 2nd ed. National Resident Matching Program; July 2018. Accessed February 28, 2020.

Osler W. Aequanimitas and Other Addresses to Medical Students, Nurses, and Practitioners of Medicine. Philadelphia P: Blakiston's Son & Co. 1914.

Palmer PJ. The Active Life: A Spirituality of Work, Creativity, and Caring. Jossey-Bass; 1999.

Rodziewicz, T. L., Houseman, B., & Hipskind, J. E. (2023). Medical Error Reduction and Prevention. In StatPearls. StatPearls Publishing.

Scott SD, Hirschinger LE, Cox KR, McCoig M, Brandt J, Hall L. The natural history of recovery for the health care provider "second victim" after adverse patient events. Qual Saf Health Care. 2009;18:325-330.

Seppälä E. Doctors who are kind have healthier patients who heal faster, according to new book. Washington Post. https://www.washingtonpost.com/lifestyle/2019/04/29/doctors-who-show-compassion-have-healthier-patients-who-heal-faster-according-new-book. Published April 29, 2019. Accessed Oct 31, 2022.

Steiner-Hofbauer V, Schrank B, Holzinger A. What is a good doctor? Wien Med Wochenschr. 2018; 168(15-16): 398-405. doi:10.1007/s10354-017-0597-8.

The Blind Men and the Elephant. Peacecorps.gov. Published 2011. Accessed September 26, 2022. https://www.peacecorps.gov/educators/resources/story-blind-men-and-elephant

Widera E, Smith A. Therapeutic Presence in the Time of COVID: Podcast with Keri Brenner and Dani Chammas. https://geripal.org/therapeutic-presence-in-time-of-covid. Published April 14, 2020.

Woods SE, Harju A, Rao S, Koo J, Kini D. (2006). Perceived biases and prejudices experienced by international medical graduates in the US post-graduate medical education system. Medical Education Online. 11(1): 4595. •

Contributors

•

Sapana Adhikari, MD
Attending Emergency Medicine Physician
Atrium Health Wake Forest Baptist
Charlotte, NC

Jazbeen Ahmad, MD
Hospitalist
Waco, TX

Sheenie Ambardar, MD
Psychiatrist, Psychotherapist, & Coach
The Happiness Psychiatrist
Los Angeles, CA

Pouya Ameli, MD, MS
Assistant Professor of Neurology and Neurosurgery
University of Florida College of Medicine
Gainesville, FL

Chinmayi Balusu
Master of Public Health Student
Department of Epidemiology
Mailman School of Public Health, Columbia University
New York, NY

Timothy J. Barreiro, DO, MPH, FCCP, FACOI, FACP
Professor of Internal Medicine
Pulmonary Health & Research Center
St. Elizabeth Health Center/Mercy Health System Youngstown
Youngstown, OH

Rohan R. Bhat
Medical Student
University of Massachusetts Chan Medical School
Worcester, MA

CONTRIBUTORS

Anna Böhler
Internal Medicine Resident
Medical University of Vienna
Vienna, Austria

Alejandra Casillas, MD, MSHS
Assistant Professor of Medicine in Residence
Division of General Internal Medicine & Health Services Research
Department of Medicine, UCLA David Geffen School of Medicine
Los Angeles, CA

Emil Chuck, PhD
Director of Advising Services
Health Professional Student Association
Huntington Beach, CA

Miriam Colleran, MB BCh BAO, MRCGP, MD, Dip_L_Q
Consultant in Palliative Medicine
St. Brigid's Hospice and Naas General Hospital
Co. Kildare, Ireland

Anna Delamerced, MD
Yale Pediatrics
New Haven, CT

Andrea Eisenberg, MD
Assistant Clinical Professor
OUWB School of Medicine, Michigan Women's Health
Bloomfield Hills, MI

Mallory Evans, BS
Oakland University William Beaumont School of Medicine
Oak Park, MI

Melissa Flanagan, LCSW
Private Practice Clinician
The Community Couch LCSW PLLC
Brooklyn, NY

Melinda Ginne, PhD
Gero-Psychologist and Behavioral Medicine Specialist
UC Berkeley Extension—Honored Instructor for Programs in Aging
Berkeley, CA

Charlotte Grinberg
Hospice Medical Director
Luminis Health Gilchrist Lifecare Institute
Annapolis, MD

Harika Kottakota, BS
Medical Student
UCLA David Geffen School of Medicine
Culver City, CA

Vincent LaBarbera, MD
Assistant Professor
Warren Alpert Medical School of Brown University
Department of Neurology
Providence, RI

Robert Lamb, PhD
Research Assistant Professor
Nature Coast Biological Station
Institute of Food and Agricultural Sciences, University of Florida
Gainesville, FL

Ajibike Lapite, MD, MPHTM
Pediatric Hematology-Oncology Fellow Physician
Texas Children's Hospital
Houston, TX

Kimberly Gronsman Lee, MD, MSc
Clinical Professor of Pediatrics
Medical University of South Carolina
Charleston, SC

Eve Louise Makoff, MD
Regional Medical Director
AltaMed PACE
Los Angeles, CA

Jeffrey Millstein, MD
Clinical Assistant Professor of Medicine
Penn Medicine
Philadelphia, PA

CONTRIBUTORS

Mayra Montalvo, MD
Assistant Professor of Neurology
University of Florida
Gainesville, FL

Audrey Nath, MD, PhD
Neurologist and Clinical Assistant Professor
University of Texas Medical Branch
Houston, TX

Chidinma Onweni, MD
Advocate Aurora Health
Milwaukee, WI

Susie Jiaxing Pan
Undergraduate Student
Boston University
Boston, MA

Amisha Patel
Medical Student
Texas A&M School of Medicine
Bryan, TX

Rachel Scheub
Medical Student
Albany Medical College
Albany, NY

Soma Sengupta, MD, PhD, MBA
Clinical Professor of Neurology
Vice Chair of Inclusive Excellence & Community Engagement
Division Chief of Neuro-Oncology, University of North Carolina
Chapel Hill, NC

Palak Shah, MD, MPH, MBA
Adjunct Faculty, Kellogg School of Management, Northwestern University
Assistant Clinical Professor
University of Arizona College of Medicine at Phoenix
Center Medical Director, Oak Street Health
Scottsdale, AZ

Blessed Sheriff, MPH
Medical Student
Brown University Warren Alpert School of Medicine
Johns Hopkins Bloomberg School of Public Health
Baltimore, MD

Zachary Simpson, BS
Medical Student
University of Oklahoma College of Medicine
Oklahoma City, OK

Maya J. Sorini, MS
Medical Student
Hackensack Meridian School of Medicine
Maywood, NJ

Danielle Wilfand
Medical Student
Case Western Reserve University
Cleveland, OH

Joanne Wilkinson, MD, MSc
Associate Professor of Family Medicine
Brown University
Providence, RI

Rebecca Lynn Williams-Karnesky, MD, PhD, MEdPsych
Endocrine Surgery Fellow
University of Wisconsin
Madison, WI

M. Daniela Orellana Zambrano, MD
University of Tennessee
Memphis, TN

Melani Zuckerman
Medical Student
Boston University Chobanian & Avedisian School of Medicine
Boston, MA •

Acknowledgements

•

Thank you to every single one of the amazing artists and writers who contributed to this book. We are honored to provide a space for your art to live. You made me cry and laugh, and oh, how did I relate. I learned so much from your experience and cumulative wisdom. Thank you to the writers whose pieces did not make the cut. Your work does not go unrecognized. I encourage all of you to keep writing, painting, drawing and expressing.

I could not have done this without the creative guidance of Ajay Major and Aleena Paul of Pager Publications. Your collaboration over the years from *in-Training* onward has inspired me and given me an irreplaceable community of expression.

I'd like to acknowledge Jonah Tower for providing feedback on the introduction and Leonid Yakhkind and Tamara Smirnova for the thoughtful discussion on these pieces from the non-medical point of view throughout the editorial process. I am grateful to everyone who taught me and shaped me to be aware of the complexities of medicine. Thank you to that group of doctors around the dinner table in Chicago—Krupa Savalia, Dania Shujjat, and Poula Ameli, to name a few—who inspired this book. I look forward to ongoing bonding over these wild careers as our journeys continue.

Sasha Yakhkind, MD •

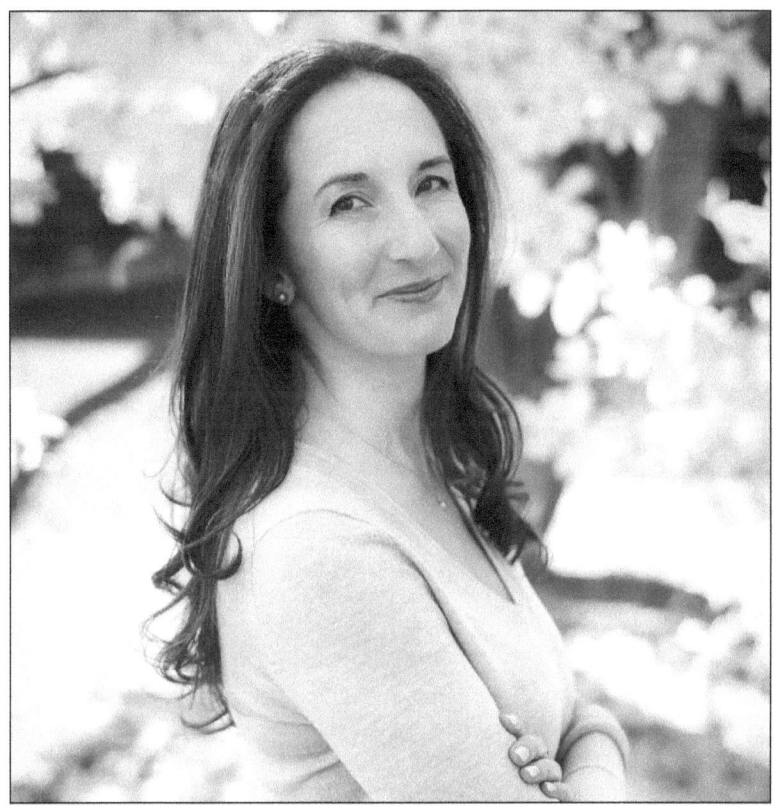

Sasha Yakhkind is a neurointensivist in her hometown of Boston. She has been a writer since her riveting (original) sequel to Jurassic Park was read out loud in front of her third grade class, and an editor since she helped run her high school newspaper. She has always found a way to stay involved in the literary community and gets a strange pleasure from deleting unnecessary commas and converting sentences to start after a single space. The days that she hasn't had time to write or read have been her hardest.

Her training has taken her from the Boston University University Professors Program to the University of South Florida SELECT program to neurology residency at Brown University and then neurocritical care fellowship at the University of Pennsylvania.

Apart from writing, she is involved in global health and health care clinician wellness initiatives at Tufts Medicine and Tufts University School of Medicine. In the neuro ICU, she loves teaching and improving care for patients with bleeding in their brains.

She spends most possible moments outdoors running, biking, on her paddle board, or cross-country skiing. Her friends will often ask where she is, as her travel bug continues to take her to far stretches of the earth.

www.ingramcontent.com/pod-product-compliance
Lightning Source LLC
Chambersburg PA
CBHW020356170426
43200CB00005B/196